[redacted]

[redacted]

TRANSLATIONAL MEDICINE

edited by
James Mittra
Christopher-Paul Milne

TRANSLATIONAL MEDICINE

THE FUTURE OF THERAPY?

PAN STANFORD PUBLISHING

Published by

Pan Stanford Publishing Pte. Ltd.
Penthouse Level, Suntec Tower 3
8 Temasek Boulevard
Singapore 038988

Email: editorial@panstanford.com
Web: www.panstanford.com

British Library Cataloguing-in-Publication Data
A catalogue record for this book is available from the British Library.

Translational Medicine: The Future of Therapy

ISBN 978-981-4316-99-6 (Hardcover)
ISBN 978-981-4364-84-3 (eBook)

Printed in the USA

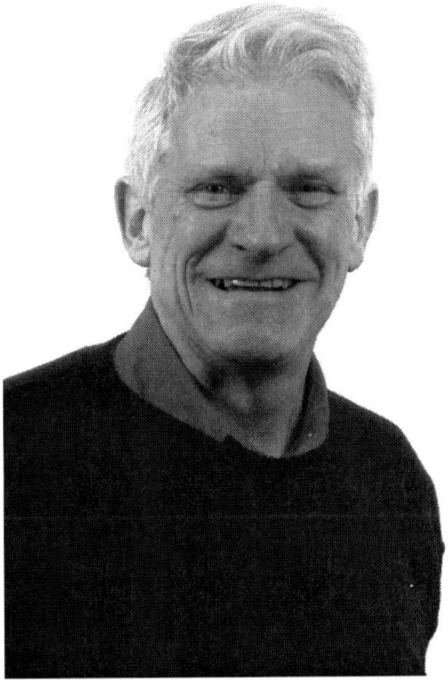

This book is dedicated to the memory of
Jim Jackson (1947–2011)

Jim Jackson was the first director and later chief executive of Alzheimer Scotland—Action on Dementia, before he decided to change career in 2008 and successfully obtained an MSc degree in translational medicine at the University of Edinburgh. Before his untimely death in 2011, Jim was conducting a doctoral study to investigate new models of evaluation for translational medicine projects, and his contribution to this book is based on his early research findings.

Contents

Preface

The opportunity to produce this book, and our motivation for editing it, emerged from a number of research synergies and joint intellectual interests between our respective institutions (the ESRC Innogen Centre at the University of Edinburgh and the Tufts Center for the Study of Drug Development), which have fermented over a number of years. With a key longstanding interest in all aspects of commercial and public-sector therapeutic innovation, we have been keen to understand the emergence and future potential of new translational processes for converting new science, technologies, and knowledge into viable clinical products and identifying potential gaps and constraints along the health innovation pathway as a whole.

In recognition of the different implications of this new translational agenda for public health policy, commercial pharmaceutical innovation and academic science, we were eager to address some of the systemic aspects of this emerging field. Rather than focus simply on the basic science and its relation to clinical practice, we felt it important to ensure the dynamic interactions of key actors and institutions in the broader healthcare sector were adequately captured. Although translational medicine (TM) has been defined, driven, and put into practice by a number of different actors at the scientific, commercial, and social/regulatory levels, the interactions between these different sectors have been an underexplored area in social and medical sciences.

Many accounts of TM tend to focus exclusively on the science and technology and often on specific disease areas, but TM is a truly interdisciplinary field in terms of its key stakeholders, working methods, and skills base. Furthermore, it encompasses much more than just basic science and clinical practice. Its success depends on the successful integration of disciplines, funding streams, collaborative research and public–private partnerships, and buy-in from regulatory bodies and policymakers. We, therefore, wanted this book to provide the first overview of TM from the perspectives of academic science, clinical practice, industry, social/regulatory systems, and social science, essentially bridging the industry, science, and society nexus.

We also sought to ensure the book was international in terms of the range of contributing authors and the scope and content of the case studies used. We were delighted with the high quality of the authors' contributions, which reflect a remarkably broad international expertise.

We hope that this book will be widely read and enjoyed by both scientists and policymakers involved in strategic decision-making around TM; social scientists interested in medical technology, innovation, and public–private partnerships; scholars interested in innovation management in the life sciences; and students now taking the increasing number of post-graduate courses in translational medicine and allied disciplines.

In addition to the contributing authors of this book, we would like to thank the publishers for their excellent guidance and work to finalize the book. We are also grateful to our respective institutions for providing us with the time to edit and contribute to this book and for funding the research that has inspired our thoughts on the subject of translational medicine and its future.

James Mittra
Christopher-Paul Milne
January 2013

Part 1

Introduction

Chapter 1

Introduction to Translational Medicine

James Mittra[a,*] and Christopher-Paul Milne[b]

[a] *ESRC Innogen Centre/STIS, University of Edinburgh, Old Surgeons' Hall, High School Yards, Edinburgh EH1 1LZ, UK*
[b] *Center for the Study of Drug Development, Tufts University Medical School, 75 Kneeland St., Suite 1100, Boston, MA 02111, USA*
*james.mittra@ed.ac.uk

Translational medicine (TM) is still a relatively new concept in the biomedical sciences, as well as the social sciences, although some of the key processes and principles underpinning it are not so novel. There has been much investment from the commercial and public sector in TM research in recent years, as pharmaceutical firms try to respond to the "productivity crisis" and high attrition rate for new therapeutic compounds [1–3] and the public sector strives to push forward its broad biomedical research agenda and build on existing evidence-based medicine to develop sustainable solutions for public health problems [4]. Successful research, development, and delivery of innovative therapies has become increasingly difficult due to a confluence of scientific, regulatory, and policy challenges. For example, of the thousands of biomarkers developed by industry and academia, only a few dozen have actually been fully validated by regulatory agencies. Few medical products that appear to be promising based on early published findings make it to the market, and fewer still become widely adopted as the standard-of-care in

Translational Medicine: The Future of Therapy
Edited by James Mittra and Christopher-Paul Milne

ISBN 978-981-4316-99-6 (Hardback), 978-981-4364-84-3 (eBook)
www.panstanford.com

the clinic. There is, in essence, a problem with the translation of new scientific knowledge into the everyday practice of medicine. Industry and the public health sector are increasingly embracing TM as a potential strategy for improving the overall health innovation cycle.

Exploiting the full potential of TM in both the public and commercial sectors often requires additional institutional models and R&D strategies from the historic "big pharma model," as well as the development and successful implementation of new organizational tools, strategies, and working methods.

In both theory and practice, TM has gained much currency over the past decade in academic medicine, the biopharmaceutical industries, and policy and regulatory communities as a means of driving forward life science innovation and ensuring it meets the continuing challenges of drug development. The hope is that it will lead to tangible benefits in terms of the production and delivery of new, safer, and more effective therapies.

However, there is continuing debate about what TM actually is and what it can realistically deliver in the short, medium, and long term. Despite enormous public and private investment in the field, TM often remains a relatively vague and ambiguous concept. This is partly a consequence of the fact that different stakeholder communities use the term in quite diverse institutional contexts, so their vision of the aims, objectives, and ultimate goals for the field can diverge quite significantly.

In this introduction we explore some of the different drivers and barriers to TM and pick out some of the most salient features that have implications for our understanding of modern health innovation. This will provide the necessary background context to the various contributions in this volume.

1.1 What Is Translational Medicine and Where Did It Come From?

The TM movement came about as a response to concern that despite the constant flow of scientific knowledge on the cellular and physiological mechanisms of many debilitating and fatal diseases, few truly novel treatments were emerging from it. This was thought to result from several root causes: clinicians in the field were not provided the opportunity to bring their clinical findings and fruitful insights to the attention of research scientists; the connections among study results from *in vitro*, *in vivo*, and *in silico* findings were not being made; and animal models and simulation programs were not sufficiently predictive of the human condition. TM really began to emerge in the broader academic and policy literature in the mid-late 1990s. In this volume, Alison Kraft talks about the tenuous relationship between lab and clinic coming to be seen by policymakers as a barrier to innovation. More specifically, there was growing concern that public investment in life science (such as the Human Genome Project) might not quickly bring about the promised economic and patient benefits. This interface between lab and clinic was therefore seen as a key area to target. Some have emphasized the seriousness of this gap as the "Valley of Death" [5].

The gap basically relates to a number of challenges facing the conventional bench-to-bedside continuum, which include various cultural, institutional, and financial barriers that underline the translation of basic research into practice and the uptake of new technologies, as well as more general challenges facing drug development, such as lack of efficacy and safety in phase 2 clinical trials, regulatory hurdles, commercial challenges, etc. Many of these gaps have been identified in a number of reports by scientists, regulatory agencies, and funders of medical research [6–10].

There was a palpable sense of urgency that translational gaps needed to be closed and translational activities to expedite the successful delivery of safe and effective therapies to patients be encouraged. However, there was still little clarity and no real consensus around the defining features of TM and its practical implementation [11].

Mario Sznol, an editorial board member of the *Journal of Translational Medicine*, suggests TM should be defined as a discipline that encompasses the following key elements [12]:

- Basic science studies which define the biological effects of therapies in humans.

- Human-centered investigations that define the biology of disease and facilitate the development of new or improved therapies.
- Non-human or non-clinical studies aimed at advancing therapies to the clinic or developing principles for the application of therapeutics to human disease.
- Any clinical trial of a therapy, emerging from the above studies, with endpoints including toxicity and/or efficacy.

In addition, in the regulatory arena:

> Translational research may be defined as appropriate product development for clinical use in various stages of investigational clinical trial. [12]

More recently, the term has come to refer more broadly to the development and use of new scientific methods and technologies, interdisciplinary approaches, and collaborative institutional arrangements to bridge the gap between basic and clinical science, exploit new science and technology in healthcare, and facilitate better exchange of knowledge, information, and expertise from "bench to bedside" *and back again*. The feedback loop from clinical practice to bench science is perhaps the most novel feature of contemporary understandings of TM and should be considered integral to any workable definition.

1.2 Different Drivers and Expectations of Translational Medicine

The definitional ambiguities around TM partly reflect the different views and expectations that key stakeholders have about the very nature of the innovation challenges and how best to meet them. The different drivers and institutional foci also reflect stakeholders' location within different innovation networks and value chains. There are three key constituencies that are driving TM.

Box 1.1 TM and the Clinical Research Community

Findings from the Human Genome Project, and the ability to selectively manipulate genes in transgenic models in mice and other species, are predicted to enhance understanding of molecular pathways of disease. These pathways can be better explored in clinical studies using modern high throughput genetic and molecular testing, complemented by state-of-the-art imaging. However, the complexity of these processes brings a risk of increasing specialization.

Some clinical researchers have embraced new basic science technologies enthusiastically, but at the expense of their training in conventional physiology and pharmacology, and in the techniques of patient-oriented research (or "experimental medicine"). Other clinical researchers feel alienated from basic science, and basic scientists may lack an appreciation of clinical research.

Academic institutions and their funding agencies have an increasing enthusiasm for exploiting commercial benefits from their research, which is most likely to be achieved by the development of ideas beyond the bench and toward the bedside, before ultimately recruiting commercial partners or investment to reach market. This requires universities and others to acquire skills and undertake research previously considered the exclusive domain of commercial companies.

Academic researchers, more so than commercial companies, are also involved in non-drug therapy, including stem cell therapy, gene therapy, etc. These activities have drawn basic scientists and academic institutions further toward clinical trial design, and this can be facilitated by the formalization of TM as a discipline.

1.2.1 *Scientific Needs/Drivers*

Scientists are embracing translational medicine to better understand and exploit the range of new technologies emerging from the life sciences, and enhance the interface between basic science and clinical medicine. Increasing sophistication at both the basic and clinical phases of biomedical innovation and delivery has led to a widening gulf between scientific researchers and clinicians. Furthermore, the complex nature of new technologies, and the subsequent need for interdisciplinary and collaborative research environments, has spurred interest in translational studies, which many believe will facilitate integrative approaches to the successful application of new tools and technologies in disease research. It is also envisaged that TM will help better define mechanisms to coordinate the quite disparate activities and knowledge domains constitutive of life science innovation and encourage research activity in neglected areas in order to complete the complementary skills mix required to deliver research from "bench to bedside" in academic and commercial settings.

1.2.2 *Commercial Needs/Drivers*

The pharmaceutical industry is currently facing a number of challenges to its conventional R&D model. There is a high attrition rate of new compounds in phase 2 clinical trials; the gap between drug discovery and development in large firms is hindering innovation and the speed of compounds through the development pathway; companies are more reliant on the knowledge and expertise of academic scientists to exploit the potential of the life sciences; and better access to patients and tissue samples is needed to improve the safety and efficacy of new drugs.

For industry, TM has taken on several meanings and consequently TM units within major pharmaceutical companies have taken various shapes in terms of scope and strategy. In some, the TM group has focused on creating a more direct connection between basic research and patient care, i.e. to better address questions related to how their drugs actually work in humans. For others, the mission has been to bridge the gap from late discovery to early clinical development so that go/no-go decisions on product candidates are now handled on a continuum rather than hands-off. For still others, the TM unit serves as the company's conduit to access outside, often experimental, R&D resources either through a consortium of research partners or academic collaborations.

Industry believes TM, and the interdisciplinary resources and expertise it encourages, will help to improve drug discovery and development processes. It is hoped that TM will help to reduce the attrition rate of compounds in phase 2 and improve the safety and efficacy of new treatments; thus meeting the increasingly strict requirements of regulators. It is envisaged that the overall costs and timescales of drug R&D will fall if translational medicine is successful. A secondary benefit may be the identification of novel drug targets. This is very much a "process-driven" approach to TM.

Box 1.2 TM and Commercial R&D

Large pre-clinical R&D divisions continue to capture new targets (some of which have been identified in academia and sometimes with clinical validation data available) and identify molecules that hit those targets. Phase 1 clinical trials often find these molecules to be safe. However, attrition in early phase 2 trials indicates that many molecules are not being found to be efficacious, using conventional indices of success. Fewer drugs are now reaching market. The worry is that many "babies are being thrown out with the bathwater" — drugs which do not meet crude criteria for success in groups of patients might actually work in a different group of patients or with a different measure of efficacy. The challenge is to give the right drug in the right amount to the right patient for the right reason. TM offers industry a method for closer interaction between R&D and clinical development groups, and between the commercial and academic sector.

Refined measurements of drug efficacy, including "biomarkers" as surrogate measures of drug interactions with their target or success in treating a disease, are being incorporated early in the R&D and clinical development pathways. Novel approaches, such as pharmacogenetics, are being used to select the right patients.

1.2.3 *Social/Regulatory Drivers*

Major concerns of regulators, politicians, and the public are the cost, safety, and efficacy of new therapeutic products. Pharmaceutical research and product development is subject to an extremely high "regulatory hurdle," which is continually changing. A variety of new genomics-based technologies are helping to identify novel compounds and improve their safety and efficacy profiles. Technology is also helping to improve the delivery of compounds to relevant disease targets.

The integration of basic and clinical knowledge and expertise early in the development pathway, through new translational processes, can be seen as an attempt to meet increased regulatory requirements and societal expectations. In particular, TM can facilitate the design and successful execution of phase 2 and phase 3 clinical trials through improvements in preclinical knowledge and understanding of drug compounds and their likely clinical effects. For example, the developing field of Stratified Medicine, which requires highly integrative and interdisciplinary research skills, is most likely to successfully progress and have a real impact on improving the safety and efficacy of new therapies through new translational processes. Furthermore, there is substantial government and charitable investment in R&D in universities and other public sector research organizations. There is a perception that rewards in terms of improvements to public health and wealth have so far been disappointing. Funding is increasingly being directed to capacity building in specific research areas, and TM has emerged as a high priority for public health-related investment.

Although there are many different drivers of TM — reflecting different stakeholder needs and expectations — there are a number of common salient features. Although many of the underlying principles and processes are not necessarily novel (the notion of bench-to-bedside long predates the emergence of TM), they have in some sense been recast and re-prioritized in new and interesting ways. What we have witnessed over the past decade is a renewed and reinvigorated research and policy agenda firmly committed to plugging gaps in the current health innovation pathway. Increasing

Box 1.3 TM and the Social/Regulatory Environment

Regulation and pricing policies, in both national and international contexts, have a significant impact on innovation processes for pharmaceuticals and the range and type of therapies successfully delivered to market. Regulation and policy can both enable and constrain innovation; often in unpredictable ways. Furthermore, social and regulatory needs and drivers for TM may not always coincide with scientific and commercial drivers. It is important to recognize the complexity of the challenges facing the different sectors, and the emerging interactions/relationships between relevant stakeholder groups, when trying to understand the development and evaluate the potential success of TM as both a new scientific discipline and organizing principle for R&D.

amounts of financial resource and research infrastructure have been built for this task. The target has been to reconceptualize the transfer of knowledge and expertise between the lab and the clinic, and to encourage the interdisciplinary and collaborative work that is considered essential if investments in life science are to translate into viable clinical therapies. This is perhaps the core of what TM is all about. There are now many experiments in TM (from basic translational projects to large scale reorganization of R&D and business models for health innovation), and attempts to meet some of the key challenges in trying to better integrate the basic science and clinical spheres [13,14].

1.3 General Aims and Scope of This Book

In recognition of the various implications of this new research trajectory for public health policy, commercial innovation, and academic science, this book addresses some of the systemic aspects of TM. Rather than focus simply on basic science and its relation to clinical practice, the collection of chapters in this volume reveal the dynamic interactions and key challenges in translating new science into viable therapies for the clinic; recognizing the crucial importance of social, commercial, and regulatory environments.

TM is being defined, driven, and put into practice by a number of different actors at the scientific, commercial, and social/regulatory levels. The interactions between these different sectors has been an under explored area in the social and medical sciences, yet they are all vital to the success of TM. Questions remain as to whether TM can actually improve the safety and efficacy of new therapies, improve delivery to patients, de-risk the clinical trials process, and lead to step-changes in regulatory protocols. There are also key issues in terms of how to evaluate TM initiatives.

The key objective of this book is to bring together the different perspectives relevant to TM and provide an overview of what TM is and how it is being put into practice. Key themes include state-of-the-art in science, technology, and clinical practice; social, scientific, commercial, and regulatory perspectives on TM; case studies of TM in both high and low resource settings; and the impact of TM on breakthrough technology and the organization of R&D. The contributors are international experts from a range of disciplines (science; medicine, science and technology studies; law, history, and innovation studies, among others), which reflects the interdisciplinary nature of the book.

Many accounts of TM tend to focus exclusively on the science and technology and are often limited to specific disease areas. However, TM is a truly interdisciplinary field in terms of its key stakeholders, working methods, and skills base. Furthermore, it encompasses much more than just basic science and clinical practice. Its success depends on the successful integration of disciplines, funding streams, collaborative research, and public–private partnerships, as well as buy-in from regulatory bodies and policymakers. In light of this, we try to provide a systemic overview of TM from "proof of concept" to delivery of therapy from the relevant stakeholder perspectives in an attempt to bridge the industry, science, and society nexus. We hope this significantly enhances conceptual and practical understanding of the emergence and progress of the field and its potential impact on basic research, therapeutic development, and future institutional infrastructure/resources.

1.4 Overview of Chapters

The book is split into four main sections. In Part 2, we have four chapters that provide in-depth discussion of some of the key drivers and broader policy context for TM. In Chapter 2, Alison Kraft nicely traces the historical underpinnings and nuances of the "translational turn" in biomedicine from the perspective of both scientists and clinicians struggling to navigate the gaps between the laboratory and the clinic, as well as the policymakers endeavoring to drive forward a new approach to biomedicine. In Chapter 3, Christopher Milne and Christine Kohn present an industry perspective on TM. The authors look at both how industry is currently exploiting translational tools, technologies, and working practices and what future directions there may be for TM in a commercial pharmaceutical context. In Chapter 4, Partha Roy (who worked until recently at the US Food and Drug Administration [FDA]) presents a regulatory perspective on TM. He explains what he considers to be the key drivers of TM and highlights some of the ways in which regulators such as the FDA can support drug development and TM processes, particularly in the context of personalized medicines and novel clinical trial design. In Chapter 5, Jim Jackson considers some of the major challenges in evaluation criteria for TM projects, which are very different in many respects to conventional biomedical research projects. Jackson begins by developing a working definition of TM before testing a new pilot evaluation model that he hopes may be developed and refined for future application in translational projects.

In Part 3, we have three papers that present the "state-of-the art" in the science and technologies underpinning TM. In Chapter 6, Robert Nussenblatt and Francis Marincola present some of the latest findings in biomarker research as it applies to improved understanding of complex biological processes, such as the treatment of cancer with biological manipulation and the biology of degenerative diseases of the eye. The authors use these examples to argue for "discovery-driven" and "hypothesis generating" human studies as a key component in TM. This presents a fundamental challenge to the current status-quo. In Chapter 7, Jingsong Wang looks specifically at non-invasive imaging biomarkers in drug development as a highly promising translational process. His chapter illustrates the current state-of-the-art and key challenges in using imaging biomarkers in clinical drug development. In Chapter 8, Indra Neil Sarkar looks at the complex and evolving field of translational bioinformatics as a key technology for bridging the traditionally segregated biological and clinical knowledge domains and respective domain-specific informatics communities. Translational bioinformatics is presented as an integrative approach that builds on focused domain-specific informatics approaches and postulates novel testable hypotheses. Sarkar provides us with an excellent overview of the different data associated with biological and clinical knowledge and the new enabling approaches that are being developed to link the two.

In Part 4, we move on to consider the institutional dynamics of TM. Two chapters provide real case examples of public–private partnerships and the organizational/institutional challenges of making them a success. In Chapter 9, James Mittra presents a case study of Scotland's Translational Medicine Research Collaboration (TMRC) to reflect on both the key opportunities and major challenges facing new collaborative models for translational science. Although TMRC is presented in this chapter as a cautionary tale, Mittra draws some useful lessons for future collaborations between the public and commercial sectors in the context of TM. In Chapter 10, Julius Mugwagwa *et al.* explore product development partnerships as a translational mechanism for delivering healthcare in low resource settings, which is often neglected in the TM literature. Looking at the International AIDS Vaccine Initiative (IAVI) as a case study, the authors highlight the challenges of healthcare delivery in the developing world and demonstrate how novel product-development partnerships (which are presented as "social technologies") can bring about effective and sustainable health care solutions.

In Part 5, we provide a broader reflection on TM as a potential exemplar for the future of therapy. Both of us rehearse some of the key thematic issues to emerge from the chapters in this book and reflect on what the future holds for TM in the context of challenges to the R&D paradigm, patient-centered healthcare, and regional geographies for innovation.

We hope that the chapters in this book provide a good, interdisciplinary overview of the key issues facing contemporary therapeutic innovation, the opportunities, and challenges posed by TM in different institutional and geographical contexts, and some evidence-based reflection on what the future is likely to hold for the field. We would like to thank all the authors for their excellent and thought-provoking contributions based on a broad range of expertise.

References

1. Tait, J., and Mittra J. (2004). Industry challenges, *Chemistry and Industry*, **6**(23) December 2004, p. 24.
2. Mittra, J. (2007). Life science innovation and the restructuring of the pharmaceutical industry: merger, acquisition and strategic alliance behaviour of large firms, *Technology Analysis and Strategic Management*, **19**(3), pp. 279–301.
3. Mittra, J. (2008). Impact of the life sciences on organisation and management of R&D in large pharmaceutical firms, *IJBT*, **10**(5), pp. 416–440.
4. *BMJ* (2008). Translational research Editorial, **337**, p. 863.
5. Butler, D. (2008). Crossing the valley of death, *Nature*, **453**, pp. 840–842.
6. FDA (2006). *Critical path opportunities report*, US Department of Health and Human Services, March, 2006.
7. Medical Research Council. (2008). *Translational research strategy*, http://www.mrc.ac.uk/consumption/groups/public/documents/content/mrc004551.pdf.
8. Cooksey, D. (2006). *A review of UK health research funding*. www.hm-treasury.gov.uk/independent_reviews/cooksey_review/cookseyreview_index.cfm.
9. Academy of Medical Sciences (2011). *A new pathway for the regulation and governance of health research*, January, 2011 (available at http://www.acmedsci.ac.uk/p99puid209.html).
10. National Institutes of Health Scientific Management Review Board (2010). *Report on translational medicine and therapeutics*. (online) Available at: http://smrb.od.nih.gov/dec/TMAT_Meeting_Formatted.pdf (accessed 3 April 2011).

11. Hait, W. (2005). Translating research into clinical practice: deliberations from the American Association for Cancer Research. *Clinical Cancer Research*, **11**(12), pp. 4275–4277.
12. Cited in Mankoff, S., *et al.* (2004). Lost in translation: obstacles to translational medicine, *Journal of Translational Medicine*, **2**(14), doi:10.1186/1479-5876-2-14.
13. Pober, J., Neuhauser, C., and Pober, J. (2001). Obstacles facing transational research in academic medical centers. *The Federation of American Societies for Experimental Biology Journal*, **15**, pp. 2303–2313.
14. Horig, H. Marincola, E., and Marincola, F. (2005). Obstacles and opportunities in translational research. *Nature Medicine*, **11**(7), pp. 705–708.

Part 2

Drivers and Barriers to Translational Medicine

Chapter 2

New Light Through an Old Window? The "Translational Turn" in Biomedical Research: A Historical Perspective

Alison Kraft
Research Fellow, Egenis, ESRC Centre for Genomics in Society, University of Exeter, Exeter, UK
a.kraft@exeter.ac.uk

2.1 Introduction

In the opening years of the 21st century the term "translation" emerged rapidly and seemingly out of nowhere as the new "buzzword" in biomedicine (Fig. 2.1). The "translational turn," evidenced in the prefixing of "translational" to — medicine, research, and science, emphasized the place of these different spheres in biomedical innovation. Embedded within the "translational turn" was the notion that all was not well with biomedical innovation and here the relationship between laboratory and clinic came in for particular criticism. The relationship between these sites has, historically, been uneasy, reflecting long-standing and deeply rooted differences between them. Constantly negotiated and renegotiated

Translational Medicine: The Future of Therapy
Edited by James Mittra and Christopher-Paul Milne

ISBN 978-981-4316-99-6 (Hardback), 978-981-4364-84-3 (eBook)
www.panstanford.com

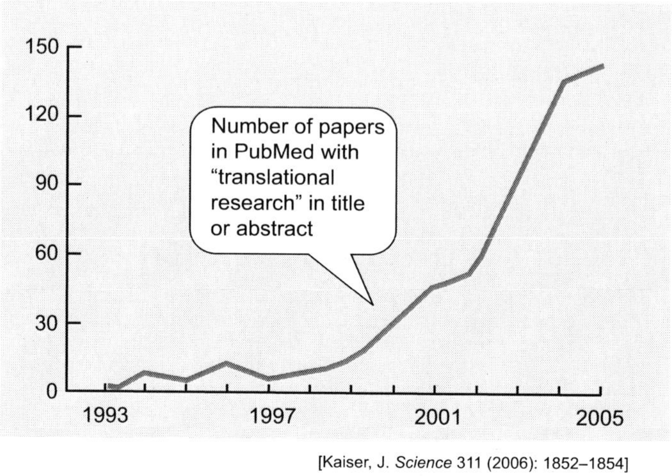

Figure 2.1 PubMed citations for "translational research," 1993–2005.

throughout the 20th century, this encounter became increasingly troubled from the 1970s onward as scientific and technical advances within molecular biology began to take practical effect in both laboratory and clinical settings. If there was agreement that problems existed, there was little agreement between practitioners in these settings about the cause(s) of these problems, or how best to solve them. In the United States, repeated warnings and misgivings from the late 1970s to the early 1990s about the relationship between the lab and the clinic, and also about the impoverished condition of clinical research, especially the patient-centred kind, went largely unheeded in policy-making circles. This was not, however, an impediment to increasing investment in biomedical research evidenced most strikingly perhaps in the rising budget of the National Institutes of Health (NIH), and the commitment in 1990 of $3bn to "biology's moonshot," the Human Genome Project (HGP). The inertia towards the lab/clinic problem created something of a policy vacuum around what many felt to be a serious and systemic problem within the biomedical enterprise — even as this continued to expand and diversify.

By the late 1990s, however, this picture looked very different. The difficulties between the lab and the clinic were being recast as a major barrier to innovation and were the subject of intense discussion within biomedical policy-making circles. The problems at the lab/clinic interface — now conceptualized as a "gap" and, moreover, one that was widening and deepening — were now perceived to be pervasive and perilous. This interface had become a "bottleneck" in the innovation process, impeding the flow of economic and patient benefits from the vast sums of public money invested in biomedical research generally and the HGP in particular. The language within policy circles was of an impending crisis: new urgency now attached to resolving the "gap" between the lab and the clinic. How could the very different worlds of the lab and the clinic be brought into closer and effective relation in order, so the reasoning went, to improve the efficiency of the (biomedical) innovation process? It was within this policy discourse that the term "translation" emerged and took on new and particular meaning. The view gained currency of "translational" work as a "bridge" between the lab and the clinic which offered a means to close the "gap"' between these sites.

Focusing primarily on developments in the United States, this chapter explores the emergence of the "translational turn," identifying the forces driving it and analyzing the debates that have attended its rise to prominence. This historical perspective compliments sociological analyses, such as those by Steven Wainwright, Clare Williams and colleagues, examining the ways in which the practice of "translational" work is reframing the ethical contours of particular fields, especially stem cell biology [1]. The chapter begins by briefly examining the long-standing difficulties that attend the relationship between science and medicine, which derive from the very different nature of clinical and laboratory work. The second section examines how these difficulties intensified after the Second World War as the biomedical enterprise expanded and came to be dominated by the concepts and techniques of molecular biology. It considers how tensions between these sites intensified as the laboratory became the primary locus of disease research and the implications of this shift for both the character of clinical research, especially clinical investigations carried out in the patient at the bedside, and the role of the physician-scientist. The chapter then discusses some of the factors that in the 1990s contributed to perceptions of a widening disconnect between the clinic and the lab, how this was increasingly conceptualized as a "gap" and how shortcomings in clinical research were recast as a "barrier" — the "rate limiting step" — in biomedical innovation. It emphasizes the 1990s as a distinctive period within biomedicine, when a convergence of several trends triggered a policy response intent on through-going reform of the biomedical enterprise, the mechanism for which was "translation." Important here were two "crises" — in clinical research and in the pharmaceutical industry. It argues that the need to realize the much-vaunted clinical potential of the HGP cast the difficulties in clinical research and at the lab/clinic interface into sharp relief and lent new urgency to tackling them. The final section focuses on the NIH *Roadmap* as a case study of a "translational" policy initiative. It analyzes the significance of this policy in giving form to the "translational" agenda in the United States and the controversies that surrounded it.

2.1.1 *Clinic and Lab: Contradictory "Spheres of Action" [2]*

> The principal criterion of success of medical practitioner — the improvement of the health of their patients — is distinct from the goals and the criteria of success of biomedical scientist. Hence, the two professions have evolved separately and often have only loose relations with each other. [3]

Writing in 1987, historian Ilana Lowy succinctly captured the fundamental differences between the world of the biomedical scientist and that of the medical practitioner, differences which have ensured that the partnership between them whilst enduring has remained uneasy. Far from new, this unease was, as Lowy noted, rooted in differences apparent since the emergence of scientific medicine in the late 19th century, a development closely associated with the growth of fields such as bacteriology and pharmacology. Maulitz has, for example, argued the importance of bacteriology in bringing about a convergence between science and medicine, evidenced in material practices such as antisepsis, whilst emphasizing too its "role as a vehicle for the infusion of the ideology of science into medicine." Characterizing the relations between science and medicine as a "contradiction between spheres of action," Maulitz also notes concerns about how scientific medicine might redefine the role and expertise of the clinician in ways that might lead away from the bedside and the patient:

> More than any other laboratory domain, bacteriology spoke to the clinician. It did so in a manner at once authoritative and paradoxical. It did not merely promise to change the way the practitioner thought about the patient's illness, it sought to ameliorate it. While it offered clinicians these new tools, it also threatened them by suggesting that scientific values, so promising of enhanced efficacy and legitimacy, might remove them from the bedside to the bench. [2]

If the potential benefits of science to medicine were clear and the model of scientific medicine compelling (efficacious treatments and therefore legitimacy), the means by which scientific insights could be brought to bear on medicine engendered several profound challenges. Never fully resolved, the contradictions and tensions between these domains remained a pressing problem throughout the 20th century, intensifying as the place of science in medicine grew ever stronger.

If, since the end of the 19th century, "scientific medicine" had engendered close relations between scientists and physicians, it had *not* made their roles identical [3]. Nor did these constituencies have shared goals and values. For example, in contrast to clinicians, the scientific community prizes the solution of scientific problems above the solution of practical problems relating to the patient in the clinical setting. Nevertheless, clinical practice and biomedical research legitimate each other. As Lowy has noted, physicians base their claim to effectiveness on scientific knowledge, whilst biomedical scientists justify the cost of their research on its potential contribution to the improvement of health [3]. The two domains were bound together in uneasy partnership as clinical investigation and scientific research came to be seen as integral to medicine. Some stunning successes were realized, evidenced most strikingly in increasing life expectancy which, for example, in the United States rose by 30 years between 1900 and 2000.

In the United States, the post-war period saw the NIH established as the single most powerful institution in US biomedicine as unprecedented levels of Federal money poured into biomedical research. Between 1945 and 1970, as its annual budget rose from $27m to $1.7bn, the NIH came to exert towering influence over US biomedical research.[a] Historically, the NIH has striven to support both clinical investigation and "basic" biomedical research, and also to foster close and productive relations between the clinic and the lab. To this end, for example, in 1952 it established a Clinical Centre in Bethesda, organized with patients on one side of the corridor and research labs on the other. For one commentator this represented "the epitome of patient-oriented research." As was emphasized at the time, the Clinical Centre would facilitate research undertaken in the patient at the bedside, providing "a means for bringing together in constant intellectual and physical contact outstanding practitioners in virtually all the clinical and laboratory specialities. This will be done in the presence of that most powerful inciter of creative thought — the sick human being for whom the vast potentialities of medical science have not yet been realized" [5].

Meanwhile, across the Atlantic, the UK Medical Research Council (MRC) was also in the 1950s restating its commitment to clinical research which it defined as "the direct study of disease in the human subject," and which it regarded as "a discipline of primary importance in any comprehensive program of research in medicine." In 1953, MRC policy in relation to clinical research was the subject of a white paper that established the MRC Clinical Research Board, responsible for oversight of a new and comprehensive research program enabled by a substantial increase in Treasury funding [6]. Although the annual budget of the MRC rose from $1.7m to $21m between 1950 and 1971, its financial resources were dwarfed by those of the NIH which fast became the largest biomedical funding agency in the world. The clear commitment to clinical research at both the MRC and the NIH was, however, no guarantee that clinical investigation would flourish, nor could it ensure close relations between the clinic and the lab and those working within these settings.

[a]Today, the NIH incorporates 27 institutes and has an annual budget of c. $29bn. Where it leads, others follow.

In the first half of the 20th century, a great deal of disease research was carried out at the bedside — by observing the patient, by keeping and analyzing meticulous records of physiological phenomena and so forth, a set of practices that for many in this period defined clinical research. Here, the patient lay at the centre of things, as the Danish physician Faber writing in 1930 noted, "clinical research must derive its inspiration from the examination of patients" [7]. In practice, clinical investigation was typically undertaken by medically trained clinicians who were also research active. Here, the clinical research function was an integral part of clinical practice. In the United States, it was the physician-scientist who fulfilled this role, widely acknowledged to form a bridge between the clinic and the lab. The patient remained at the centre of the physician-scientist's work, a dynamic captured by M. J. Shear in 1951: "In our own time, the majority of advances in understanding human physiology came from research on patients, and particularly in the United States, the physician-scientists became the paradigm" [8]. Shear went on to note that, whilst the key role of the physician-scientist provided for a flow of information from bedside to the laboratory this was, in practice, matched by both research and close collaboration with those based in the laboratory. Put simply, the physician-scientist role helped to keep the patient centre-stage and to integrate science and medicine thereby easing some of the contradictions between the clinic and the lab.

2.2 Bridging Clinic and Lab: The Physician-Scientist

> Some referred to me as a basic scientist because I worked in the laboratory, asked about mechanisms of disease, and employed reductionist approaches. But I always thought of myself as a clinical investigator, because the inspiration for the work always came from caring for sick children and because much of the work was carried out with intact patients and their families. [9]

The recollections of Leon Rosenberg, whose career as a physician-scientist spanned 40 years from the 1960s, give some sense of the duality of this distinctive role. Qualified as medical practitioners and typically holding a PhD, the physician-scientist was able — by training, experience and outlook — to function effectively in a dual role combining clinical practice with research at the bedside and/or in the laboratory. For Lowy, physician-scientists were "... able to bridge, at least partially the gap between the biological mode of thought and the medical one, and produced a situation in which practical medical questions were able to influence directly biomedical research" [3]. They facilitated a flow of information from bedside-to-bench through which clinical observation/investigation could feedback into and shape laboratory research. In the course of Rosenberg's career, however, this dual role became increasingly difficult to sustain not least amid the profound changes wrought by molecular biology. Some sense of the magnitude of these changes, and of concerns raised about them at the time, are apparent in an address by Donald Seldin, President of the American Society for Clinical Investigation, at the Society's 58th Annual Meeting in 1966:

> ... the widespread application to biologic systems of the methods and theories of the generalizing sciences, physics and chemistry, has reshaped medicine. The most dramatic manifestation of this, perhaps, is the enormous increase in diagnostic and therapeutic tools available for the management of disease.... Perhaps even more important than these technologic triumphs was the growth of medical science itself. Powerful predictive and explanatory theories were elaborated. Whole new areas of medicine were developed.... In a real sense, medicine was transformed from a crude empirical discipline into a scientific enterprise of formidable sophistication and power. [10]

The thrust of Seldin's address concerned the impact of the changing character of what was increasingly referred to as biomedical research on the dual role of the physician-scientist. In particular, he wondered whether it was possible for one person to give sufficient time to both the patient and to research. Seldin warned against the emergence of "two classes of clinician" — one responsible for the clinical care of patients and the other whose primary concern was that of research. Emphasizing that biomedical research should not become isolated from clinical investigation, he urged the creation of conditions in which the dual role of the physician-scientist could be maintained and, ideally, flourish. Yet, in the ensuing decades, the trends identified by Seldin intensified. Centrally implicated in this was the growing power of molecular biology, which engendered a shift in which disease research became increasingly the province of the laboratory and of experts other than practicing clinicians. Whilst molecular biology flourished as resources flowed into the laboratory, research centred on the whole patient in the clinical setting (clinical investigation) by contrast, began to flounder.

2.2.1 *Molecular Biology: Ascendancy of Lab*

Evelyn Fox Keller defined molecular biology in terms of three conceptual shifts: the relocation of life into the gene; the redefinition of life into the genetic code; and the recasting of the goals of biological science towards the "effective mastery over the processes of making and remaking life" [11]. These shifts took place in parallel and were interdependent. They resulted in an intensification of experimentalism within biology which, in her view, conferred a new status and authority on this field. Molecular biology constituted a new approach to biology and Lily Kay captures the diffuse character of this "new biology" in her description of it as a "disciplinary trend" synonymous with the laboratory. Here, life and disease processes were studied at the molecular level using an ever-expanding array of sophisticated technologies [12]. Laden with the kudos of the scientific laboratory and its approaches, molecular biology was perceived as "cutting edge" science which, in claims to discern the fundamental causes of disease, promised novel pathways to enhanced treatments for disease. Although the term was first coined by Warren Weaver in 1938, for Bruno Strasser molecular biology "acquired a social reality only around 1960" [13]. It was in the ensuing decades that the success of molecular biology began to change the kind of work done in the lab and the clinic and reconfigure the balance of power between them.

In association with these developments there emerged a new "biomedical" paradigm, a hybrid term articulating the ever-closer interplay between biology and medicine, which both defined a new biomedical model of the body and provided the intellectual framework within which the molecular "vision" of life flourished. Within the biomedical paradigm, attention focused on the molecular basis of disease. In this avowedly reductionist approach, the pathological process was seen to reside in faulty molecules, typically defective proteins and, later, genes. The concept of "molecular disease" was first given form in 1949 with the publication by Linus Pauling *et al* of a paper identifying the molecular mechanism underlying sickle cell anaemia — a fault in the haemoglobin component of red blood cells [14, 15]. The two decades following Pauling's paper saw genetics become a dominant force within molecular biology with the elucidation in 1953 of the structure of DNA and the unravelling of the genetic mechanism and the deciphering of the genetic code by 1966. By 1957, the "cause" of sickle cell anaemia was recast in genetic terms. It was now understood to result from a fault in the gene coding for the constituent amino acids of haemoglobin. The view that disease resided in DNA rapidly gained currency and over the next two decades was encapsulated in the notion of "genetic disease," a concept which, in Fox Keller's view, served also to emancipate medical genetics from its association with eugenics, paving the way for the rehabilitation of human genetics [16].

Molecular biology proved hugely successful, as evidenced by the inception of new journals, such as the *Journal of Molecular Biology* (1959), the creation of laboratories, such as the Laboratory for Molecular Biology in Cambridge, United Kingdom, and the European Molecular Biology Organization (1963) and the establishment of courses, lectureships, and research posts within universities [17,13]. Its expansion and institutional success was made possible by strong support from national funding bodies, notably the NIH in the United States and the MRC in the United Kingdom. This at a time when in the United States and across Europe, unprecedented levels of state funding were channelled into biomedical research generally. The success of molecular biology engendered a trend in which those undertaking research into diseases were drawn increasingly to the laboratory bench. Resources within biology were gravitating to the molecular biology laboratory where biomedicine was given form and meaning.

Molecular biology transformed the study of disease and made the laboratory the locus of disease research. Its dominance also fuelled an interpretation of the dynamic between the lab and the clinic as one in which, predominantly, information flowed from bench to bedside [18]. In other words, it fostered a one-way "linear" model of biomedical innovation in which the bench was pre-eminent.[b] This model was fiercely contested not least by clinicians who argued forcefully that clinical observation and investigation could make vital contributions to understanding disease, had a central role to play in bringing about medical and scientific advances and that, as such, ought to be valued and funded. However, by the 1970s, those expressing such views were battling in difficult circumstances as, in contrast to the success and growing power of molecular biology, the role of the physician-scientist grew more difficult, with far-reaching implications for patient-centred clinical investigation.

2.3 The Physician-Scientist: An "Endangered Species"?

By the 1970s, the role of the physician-scientist was becoming unsustainable. In addition to the dynamics noted above, the perception grew that clinical investigation was unattractive, inherently difficult, of low status and, some claimed, relatively poorly remunerated. Clinical research of the patient-centred kind was inherently "messy" and its outcomes less predictable in terms, for example, of yielding research publications, an important consideration when building a research career and in the competition to secure research funding. A sharp contrast could be drawn with a career in molecular biological research, as summarized in a 1998 review:

> During the past thirty years, the capacity to study mechanism of cell function at the molecular level has understandably shifted the attention of the majority of biomedical scientists away from an

[b]For a discussion of how biomedicine was seen to fuel a 'bench to bedside' linear account of biomedical innovation see: Keating, P., and Cambrosio, A., Does biomedicine entail the successful reduction of pathology to biology?, *Perspectives in Biology and Medicine* 47/3 (2004), pp. 357–371.

> analysis of the "whole animal" and toward a more manageable and often more productive studies of the function of isolated cells and genes. [19]

Perhaps unsurprisingly, increasing numbers were attracted into the laboratory and to careers conducting disease research in molecular biology which offered advantages in terms of remuneration, career pathway, and status. The ranks of the physician-scientist began to dwindle. Raising the alarm about this in the *NEJM* in 1979, James Wyngaarden also highlighted patterns of NIH funding in the preceding decade or so, in which it was apparent that laboratory-based researchers were, to a considerable extent, outstripping physician-scientists (clinical investigators) [20]. Critics pointed to this as evidence that NIH funding for biomedical research was weighted heavily towards molecular biology and laboratory-based studies. Wyngaarden, later a director of the NIH, triggered a highly charged debate which exposed the long-standing tensions between clinic and lab-based researchers as each now sought to defend and promote their respective agendas.

With hindsight, those arguing the cause of the physician-scientist and seeking to rectify what they felt to be the impoverished condition of clinical investigation were, by the late 1980s, fighting a rearguard action. In the United States, Gordon Gill galvanized the debate with a provocative article entitled "The end of the physician-scientist" in which he argued that many "had been seduced by the power of molecular biology and had abandoned patient-oriented research" [21]. Many were worried about the vacuum they saw forming in which biological problems — those detected in the patient at the bedside — were increasingly overlooked. In effect, the fears expressed by Seldin in 1966 had become a reality. Clinical practice and investigation were increasingly separated from the research function and whilst some clinicians continued with clinical investigation in the patient at the bedside, many others pursued a different kind of clinical research in the laboratory. In the United States, some viewed the situation in clinical investigation as so dire and the implications so grave that they began to talk in terms of an approaching crisis.

2.3.1 *The 1990s: Two Crises . . . and a "Moonshot"*

The 1990s were a turbulent period within US biomedicine. Between 1993 and 2001, the Clinton administration authorized a vast expansion in NIH funds, including a doubling of support in the 5-year period beginning in 1998 (from $13.6bn to over $27bn). With this came expectations of practical returns on this investment, yet key parts of the increasingly vast and complex "ecosystem" through which these returns would be delivered were considered by many to be in crisis. Certainly, many were of the view that clinical research was not functioning effectively. Elsewhere, serious problems were becoming apparent in the pharmaceutical industry. Although the number of new drugs launched annually had been falling steadily since the 1970s, the continued downturn in the 1990s, together with thinning product pipelines and, as companies emphasized, the escalating costs of drug innovation, were interpreted by many as evidence that the industry was facing an acute "productivity" crisis. The HGP was therefore especially welcomed by the pharmaceutical industry which, as Kubinyi has noted, "eagerly awaited its results, expecting a myriad of promising new targets" [22]. If the implications for biomedical innovation of the long-standing difficulties in clinical research and pharmaceutical innovation had been the subject of on-going discussion, the HGP brought the question of efficiency into much sharper focus. As the project approached completion, a rhetoric emerged within policy circles of a need to create conditions and structures within which the founding vision of the HGP — as a therapeutic panacea — could best be realized. Here, the efficiency of clinical research and the relations between the lab and the clinic would be critical in enabling the pharmaceutical industry to develop new products from "druggable targets" identified by the HGP.

By the mid-1990s, it was already apparent that rendering the genome sequence clinically useful would be much more difficult than initially envisaged. The stakes were very high. At a cost of approximately $3bn and given the "hype and hope" that had surrounded the project's inception, a return on this investment was essential. Arguably, the HGP stood as a test of the credibility of the biomedical paradigm, including molecular biology and genetics. A theme emerged that the infrastructure of the biomedical enterprise might be ill-equipped to meet the challenge of realizing the founding vision of the HGP. This shaped the on-going debate about the problems in clinical research and at the lab/clinic interface, which came to be described as "barriers" and "bottlenecks" impeding the innovation process. In policy circles, the language became that of overhauling the structures, practices, and culture within those institutions involved in biomedical research/innovation to overcome these barriers and bottlenecks. The emphasis on "translation" provided one means by which this process was begun.

2.3.1.1 The crisis in clinical research

> What appeared to be an endangering of clinical investigation in the late 1970s has become a serious crisis today. This crisis could lead to failure of an enterprise and limitation of potential advancements of clinical research in the next millennium. The entire "ecosystem" of clinical research is in danger of extinction. [23]

The views of Thompson and Moskowitz exemplified the concerns of many in the United States in the late 1990s regarding what they saw to be a growing crisis in clinical research [24]. Though not all clinical research was in difficulty — the pattern varied across institutions, regions, and specialisms — there was nevertheless a gathering sense of clinical research as "embattled." The eyes of all commentators were firmly fixed on the future. Restating arguments first voiced in the 1960s and 1970s, many emphasized the importance in that future of clinical investigation focused on the "whole patient." Writing in 1995, Barbara Culliton argued clinical investigation to be an "endangered science" and that policy-makers had been "lulled into" thinking that basic science had supplanted the need to study patients. In her view, realizing clinical advances from molecular biology and the HGP would require exactly this kind of clinical research [4]. The capacity for this had, as many noted, been eroded by the dwindling ranks of the physician-scientist, whose opportunities for clinical investigation were, in Culliton's view, also being adversely affected at this time by economically driven healthcare reforms which were "about money, not health." In 1997, the "clinical investigator" — a role associated with the physician-scientist — was, according to Goldstein and Brown, "bewitched, bothered and bewildered" [25].

It is clear too that many laid the blame for the crisis in clinical investigation in no small part at the door of the NIH. A figure commonly cited was that the NIH devoted just 33% of its budget to clinical research. In 1994, an Institute of Medicine Report drew attention to declining rates of NIH support for clinical research, fuelling charges that its "indifference" to it underpinned the growing imbalance between clinical and laboratory-based research, a trend first identified by Wyngaarden in 1979 [26]. The mood did not pass unnoticed at the NIH which launched its own enquiries into the matter. In 1995, then director Harold Varmus convened a Director's Panel on clinical research, later named the Clinical Research Panel (Nathan Committee), to look into the problems of clinical research. Reporting in 1997/8, the Nathan Committee moved first to deny charges of an imbalance in the distribution by the NIH of funds for clinical and lab-based research and emphasized the need for both kinds of work, including the "continued production of useful clinical research that can be rapidly applied for the benefit of our patients, the taxpayers who fund the research in the first place" [27]. Undoubtedly with an eye to the completion of the HGP — an NIH sponsored enterprise — the Nathan Committee also emphasized that medicine stood at a distinctive moment in its history:

> We are in the midst of a critical period in medicine. The promise of a future in which advances in basic biomedical research can lead to improved diagnosis and therapy is threatened by a loss of confidence on the part of clinical investigators and the future of medicine requires success in clinical medicine. [27]

Whilst Nathan acknowledged that reform was needed, the question as to its form and extent remained unclear. If clinical research was to be reformed, then its definition would be crucial. However, there was little agreement on its meaning. It had long been a slippery term encompassing a range of diverse activities, from patient-centred research at the bedside, to lab-based research into the molecular basis of disease, to the clinical trial. It was here that the Nathan Committee ignited fiercest debate [28]. To the chagrin of many, Nathan defined clinical research very broadly, and included activities such as the development of new technologies and lab-based studies of the mechanisms of human disease. Many rejected this definition, arguing that clinical research should not include testing new drugs, devices, and techniques in patients, but rather should encompass clinical investigation at the bedside in the patient. As one commentator later put it "real clinical science ought not to be conflated with the mere testing of technologies (including drugs) nor with outcomes research" [29]. The definition of clinical research mattered enormously to all those involved and the debate about it was lively and protracted.

The Nathan Committee provides a window onto thinking within senior biomedical policy circles in the late 1990s and within its findings it is possible to discern themes and shifts important in creating a context for the formulation of and emerging emphasis on "translation." In its findings, clinical research was recast as a barrier to moving scientific advances into the clinic, whilst innovation was identified much more strongly as the primary goal of all parts of the biomedical enterprise. Furthermore, it is in this and other policy documents concerned with the problems facing clinical research that a rhetoric of utility and patient benefit emerges strongly, coupled to an emphasis on the patient as tax-payer. Perhaps this reflected the ever-greater emphasis within biomedical and healthcare policy circles in the 1990s on ensuring a return on investment, which saw accountability and a "value-for-money" ethos feature more explicitly in the research funding system. This was apparent in a report from the influential Institute of Medicine (IoM) Clinical Research Roundtable in 2000 which, again emphasizing the distinctiveness of the moment, concluded:

> The US is at a decisive point in its investment in biomedical research and the nation's health. The scientific revolutions in biology, chemistry and physics during the past century, combined with the more recent doubling of the NIH budget and sequencing of the human genome, now combine to set the stage for a dramatic alleviation of human suffering from disease. [30]

Like Nathan before it, "translation" featured prominently in this report, which identified a number of what it called "translational blocks" impeding the clinical research enterprise that must be addressed to improve performance. It was in these reports that the terms "translation" and "translational research" gained currency as a means to articulate the aspirations within policy circles of overcoming "barriers" to innovation. In a double movement, translation served as a mechanism for improving efficiency whilst also reorienting biomedical research more strongly towards the goals of innovation and utility. The rationale for reform was animated by concerns to reap clinical advances from the HGP whilst being strongly shaped by economic considerations. A rhetoric that emphasized an economic "ethic" (a return on investment for the tax payer) and a welfare "ethic" (delivering patient (tax payer) benefit) smoothed political difficulties and resonated with the public. Reform seemed desirable and legitimate in order to equip the system to meet the (anticipated) demands of biomedical innovation in the post-genomic era.

2.3.1.2 The crisis in the pharmaceutical industry

Meanwhile, in another part of the biomedical enterprise, the pharmaceutical industry was encountering a different set of problems. Having diversified from its post-war reliance on antibiotics, the focus within the industry lay firmly with the chronic, prevalent diseases afflicting western societies, notably cardiovascular disease, cancer, and mental illness. For these complex conditions the industry adopted an approach referred to as rational drug design. Here, physiological processes were interpreted in molecular terms. Drugs were synthesized chemically and designed to target — to mimic, block, or modulate — a particular molecular structure; for example, an enzyme or cell receptor, associated with a disease process. The anti-hypertensive drug *Captopril* launched in 1977 by Bristol Myers Squibb is generally considered to be the first drug of this kind to reach the market, and was made possible by new understandings of the role of calcium ions in hypertension. Eclipsing diuretics, the previous drug of choice for hypertension, one commentator described rational drug design as marking a "true technological

Table 2.1 New drugs launched in 1951–1975

Period	Average no. of new drugs/year (US)
1951–1954	39
1955–1958	42
1959–1962	46
1963–1966	17
1967–1970	15
1971–1975	15

Source: Bognor, W. C., *Drugs to Market* (1996), p. 95.

revolution in drug development" [31]. Certainly, it engendered a cognitive shift to a more theory-driven approach to drug discovery and design — made possible by the study of disease at the molecular level. However, as is clear from Table 2.1, for all its success, the number of new drugs launched each year by the industry fell steadily from the 1960s whilst the cost of bringing a drug to market rose sharply.

As is clear from Fig. 2.2, sharply rising research and developments costs within the industry were not accompanied by an increase in the number of new drugs launched annually, a situation

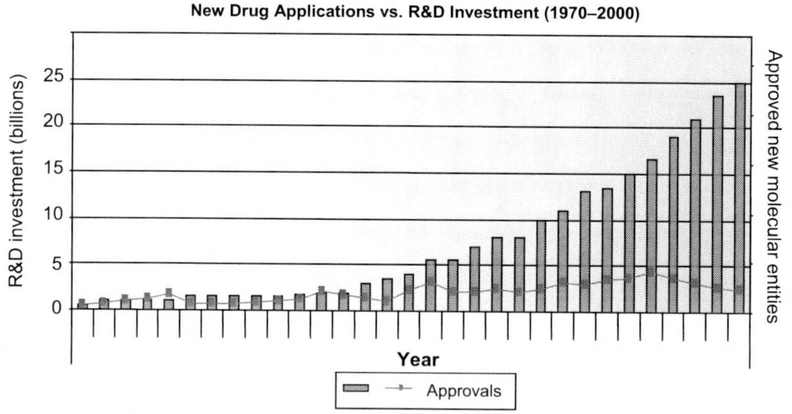

Figure 2.2 New drug applications versus R&D expenditure, 1970–2000 (Source: Schmid, E., and Smith, D. A. (2004). Is pharmaceutical R&D just a game of chance or can strategy make a difference?, *Drug Discovery Today*, 9, pp. 18–26).

that triggered talk of a "productivity crisis." For the first time, the main channel through which the biomedical enterprise delivered on its therapeutic potential — pharmaceuticals, and the industry which had flourished around this form of medical intervention — appeared to some to be in serious difficulty.

However, a new approach to drug innovation was to emerge from advances within molecular biology that also gave rise to a new commercial sector, that of biotechnology. Writing in 1986, Susan Wright argued that, by the mid-1970s, the "technical and social characteristics" of molecular biology had reached a point where the field was "ripe" for practical application, realized with the development in the mid-1970s of recombinant-DNA (rDNA) technology [32]. rDNA transformed the hitherto esoteric field of molecular biology in numerous ways. Its practical applications made possible the large-scale production of virtually any protein of known amino-acid sequence. Initially a revolution in drug manufacturing, the rDNA technique was used to generate therapeutic replacement proteins, such as (human) insulin, first launched under the brand name *Humulin* in 1982 by the biotechnology company Genentech in collaboration with Eli Lilly. Although this new class of "biopharmaceutical" was to become an important part of the pharmaceutical arsenal, the new biotechnological route to drug innovation failed to counteract the downward trend in the number of new drugs launched annually.

The advent of rDNA and other biotechnological techniques did, however, mark the beginning of a new and different era within molecular biology. The life sciences became to a much greater extent an applied and commercially oriented scientific field [33]. A vast expansion of intellectual property followed the award in 1980 to Cohen and Boyer of a patent on the rDNA technique and the Bayh-Dole Act of the same year. In turn, these developments engendered fundamental alterations in the practices, organization, and goals/priorities of the biological sciences in which, as Daniel Kleinman has put it, "... a broad commitment to sharing in the name of scientific advance has been largely displaced by a commitment to private property associated with the development of the biotechnology industry" [34].

It was around this time that James Wyngaarden first drew attention to the ailing condition of the physician-scientist and clinical investigation. As UK commentator John Bell observed, the 1970s marked a turning point in which an increasing emphasis on the molecular and genetic-basis of disease shifted research away from the bedside to the laboratory. As he put it, "the surge in activity in molecular science has led to a substantial reduction in both research and researchers in clinical science" [35]. As Barbara Culliton ruefully observed in 1995:

> The molecular revolution, ushered in with the discovery of rDNA techniques in the early 1970s, has enabled scientists to make astonishing discoveries about the functions of genes and molecules without examination. The researcher with a PhD degree and substantial training in molecular biology became a major player in biomedical science, sometimes overshadowing the physician-scientist. But in the final analysis, the fruits of molecular research must still be tested on living patients and for this, the physician-scientist remains essential. [4]

Culliton argued that whatever advances derived from molecular biology, either in terms of understanding disease or in the development of new drugs, the value of these "fruits" could only be assessed in the patient, where clinical investigation and the skills of the physician-scientist were essential. Strategically, some physician-scientists began to emphasize the importance of clinical investigation for realizing the medical potential of the HGP:

> When we have mapped and sequenced the entire human genome, who is going to make the long-sought connections between these genes and sick people if there are no physicians engaged in answering tomorrow's questions about the role that genes play in virtually all medical problems. [9]

By this time, the HGP was uppermost in the minds of many involved in biomedical and clinical research, not least because of the demands its completion might place on the practices, organization, and institutions of the biomedical enterprise and how these might be changed by it.

2.3.1.3 The human genome project: "biology's moonshot"

The HGP symbolized and legitimated the power and authority of molecular biology, consolidated the dominance of genetic-based understandings of disease, and promised a new chapter in drug innovation. As already noted, the concept of genetic disease gained currency during the 1980s and, in Fox Keller's view, by emancipating medical genetics from its tainted association with eugenics contributed substantially to a climate by the end of that decade in which the HGP appeared both "reasonable and desirable" [16]. By this time too, the technical prowess that was one hallmark of molecular biology rendered the sequencing of the human genome possible. Nevertheless, the decision to fund the HGP, taken under George Bush senior, was contested and politicized. As Daniel Kevles has shown, the project — a joint enterprise between the Department of Energy and the NIH and animated in part by a concern to maintain US leadership in biotechnology — was controversial in two key respects. Within biology, there was criticism of its avowedly reductionist ("genocentric") character; some saw it as "bad science" which, in its reliance on automated technology, would consign the biologist to a life of "gene drudgery" [36]. Secondly, the HGP was not the only large-scale scientific project for which funding was being sought and the competition was fierce. That funding was secured for the HGP rested in no small part on its much-vaunted therapeutic promise and its commercial potential. Its first director, James D. Watson, envisaged that the genome sequence would "not only help us understand how we function as healthy human beings, but will also explain at the chemical level, the role of genetic factors in a multitude of diseases, such as cancer, Alzheimer's disease, and schizophrenia, that diminish the lives of so many people" [37].

From the outset, a great deal was riding on the HGP. It stood as a test of the reductionist paradigms of molecular biology and genetic disease, and of the relevance of these for treating human disease. The credibility of those who had "backed" this project was also at stake, including the NIH and the US government. Perhaps because of the extravagant "hype" surrounding its inception and which continued as it was underway, there was also widespread public expectation that new insights derived from the HGP would readily yield benefits for patients. The pharmaceutical industry had a vested interest in the HGP, seeing in it a potential solution to its productivity "crisis" in that it would provide a wealth of new "targets" which could serve as a starting point in drug innovation. This vision was captured in a model of innovation that proceeded in linear fashion from "gene-to-drug," around which a small but vibrant genomics sector flourished in the early 1990s.

By the mid-1990s, however, it was apparent that realizing the founding visions of the HGP would take much longer than initially hoped. Rendering the genome clinically useful was a much more complex and time-consuming process wholly reliant upon new specialist fields such as bioinformatics ("a platform" to fight all kinds of diseases), new interdisciplinary forms of expertise and new technologies, such as high throughput screening [22]. The genomics sector floundered as the inadequacy of the "gene-to-drug" vision undercut hopes of emulating the success of the biotechnology sector two decades earlier [38]. This did not diminish the unbridled optimism with which the completion of the first draft of the genome sequence in June 2000 was met by President Bill Clinton and British Prime Minister, Tony Blair, who spoke enthusiastically of "a breakthrough that opens the way for massive advances in the treatment of cancer and hereditary diseases" which took "humankind across a frontier and into a new era" (Tony Blair, 26.6.2000). The rhetoric of beginnings and breakthroughs, of eradicating cancer in particular, and of revolutionizing healthcare belied the daunting realities. Practical clinical benefit remained distant possibilities: the draft sequence was, in effect, only the beginning. Bringing the project to fruition in the sense of effective therapies for those diseases foregrounded by Clinton and Blair would require a great deal more research and a further investment of public funds. It would also require addressing the problems of clinical research and the lab/clinic interface.

Within a year of the completion of the first draft of the human genome, George Bush (junior) succeeded Bill Clinton in the White House. The fiscally prudent Bush was now looking for returns on past investment in biomedical research, whilst pegging NIH funding at the levels set by his predecessor. Following protocol, Bush appointed a new director of the NIH and his choice of an

NIH outsider, Elias Zerhouni of Johns Hopkins University, signalled change. A physician-scientist specializing in radiology, Zerhouni had a track record both as a business entrepreneur (through his involvement in a number of medical technology companies) and a reform-minded administrator. As a physician-scientist, he was well-placed to understand the difficulties in clinical investigation and was also, perhaps, especially motivated to "rebalance" the funding portfolio of the NIH. On appointment in May 2002, Zerhouni immediately undertook a wide-ranging review of NIH policy, including its support of/provision for clinical investigation, engaging at "grass roots" level to identify "roadblocks" to research and to formulate future policy priorities. The findings provided the basis for a policy known as *The Roadmap.* This initiative gave meaning and form to the term "translational" research and also became perhaps the defining feature of Zerhouni's 6-year term as NIH director. Through the mechanism of "translational research," the *Roadmap* sought to reform core components of the US biomedical research enterprise to reflect what he called the "new reality" of the post-genomic era [39].

2.3.1.4 The "translational turn": meaning(s) from policy?

> The NIH is at a critical moment in its prestigious history. As the 21st century unfolds, discovery in the life sciences is accelerating at an unprecedented rate. Although the sequencing of the human genome presents vast opportunities for researchers, it also creates a series of challenges that will redefine the ways that medical research is conducted and, ultimately, how research leads to improvements in health. [39]

The NIH *Roadmap* articulated an avowedly "translational" agenda. It gave meaning and form to the use of the term within policy reports such as those of the Nathan Committee and the IoM. As its architect, Zerhouni saw the *Roadmap* as a means to "transform the way the biomedical giant in Bethesda does business." It was also fundamentally about bringing insights from the HGP to bear on clinical practice, that is, to realize its much-vaunted therapeutic potential. Unveiled in October 2003, the *Roadmap* budget was set at $2.1bn over 6 years, a staggering amount by European standards but, in NIH terms relatively modest, representing 1.7% of the total NIH annual budget in 2003.[c]

In explaining and promoting the *Roadmap*, Zerhouni routinely emphasized that the NIH stood at a decisive moment in its history — a position he linked to the HGP. For him, the future of both was entwined. It might also, in part, be interpreted as a response to the criticisms laid at its door by Wyngaarden in 1979 and others since, including Alan Schechter who in 1998 had reminded the NIH that it was firstly a "health agency" [28]. Certainly, some saw the *Roadmap* as a revitalization strategy for the NIH through which it might reassert its leadership in biomedical research, within the United States and beyond. By the time Zerhouni arrived at the NIH, it was clear that the genome sequence raised many more questions than it answered. In addressing the "gap" between genomic data and medicine, the task was twofold. It required both more understanding of complex biology and the development of pathways to facilitate the effective transfer of this science into the clinic. Central to this was clinical research which, as will be recalled, was beset with serious and long-standing difficulties. It was to these issues that the *Roadmap* spoke and it did so using the mantra of translation.

Organized into three programs, the *Roadmap* was targeted to those areas considered most directly relevant to realizing the therapeutic potential long-imputed to the HGP — clinical research, drug discovery, and the development of inter-disciplinarity (Table 2.2). The "New Pathways to Discovery" program spoke to the pharmaceutical industry. The "Re-engineering of the Clinical Research Enterprise" program engaged with the long-standing difficulties in clinical research, establishing translational research centres that would bring together the diverse range of expertise found at the lab/clinic interface. Significantly and controversially, this encompassed the clinical trial: in this move, clinical research also became much more strongly oriented to clinical trial-related

[c]In 2003, the NIH budget for clinical research stood at $8.4bn, representing c. 33% of the total NIH annual budget.

Table 2.2 The NIH Roadmap — key programs [39]

Program	$m FY 2004	Summary of key elements
New pathways to discovery	64.1	Includes a library of 500,000 small molecules; technologies to study protein interactions; establishment of biocomputing and nanomedicine centres.
Re-engineering the clinical research enterprise	37.6	Translational research centres; harmonization of regulations; integrated clinical networks; standardized national clinical trials data system; clinical training awards to build a cadre of community physicians trained in clinical research.
Research teams of the future	26.6	NIH Director's Innovator Awards (5 years, based on "creative potential"); interdisciplinary research centres; training awards; public–private liaison.

activities. The "Research Teams of the Future" program sought to foster interdisciplinary approaches to innovation. Underlying all programs was an ethos supportive of the view that clinical insights had a role to play in shaping "basic" research. Overall, the *Roadmap* sought to build stronger integration of and collaboration between all participating constituencies in the innovation process.

Zerhouni defended the *Roadmap* with a rhetoric that emphasized the need to engage with the "new realities," which required more tools, cross-disciplinary teams, and an overhaul of the infrastructure for clinical trials. As he argued, it provided a way of "synergizing areas that no institute either has the mission or resources to invest in." For him, the *Roadmap* was setting out a process to establish translational research as the new paradigm in biomedical research — which would foster the alignment of all constituencies within the innovation process, to develop "sustainable and integrated efforts in translational and clinical research that can yield new products, approaches, and diagnostic tools in an efficient seamless, manner" [39]. He saw this as the basis for realizing a "new vision of health care" based on improved molecular understanding of diseases in the wake of the HGP and from fields such as genomics, proteomics, and bio-imaging [40]. The initiative was at once programmatic and pragmatic, seeking to address two interwoven "gaps": that between the sequence of the human genome and its usefulness in the clinical setting, and that existing between the lab and the clinic.

The *Roadmap* and the drive to install "translational research" as an ideal model of biomedical work elicited various responses. Figure 2.1 suggests its ready adoption in the literature, whilst in 2006, in a striking endorsement of the translational turn, the *Journal of Laboratory and Clinical Medicine* established in the 1920s changed its name to *Translational Research.* Elsewhere, the response to the *Roadmap* and the model of "translational research" embedded within it was somewhat less enthusiastic; it drew criticism from several quarters. Some objected, in principle, to what they saw as an overly interventionist, draconian, "top down" initiative. There was an especially vehement backlash from within the "basic" research community, which saw in it a move away from the NIH's historically strong support for "basic" research. Gerald Weissman, editor of the journal of the Federation of American Societies for Experimental Biology (FASEB) derided the policy as part of his wider hostility to "protocols from above directing (our) science" and of the prevailing culture within US science in which "childish curiosity" — the root of all good science — is more likely to be bent to the service of politics than to human needs" [41]. Others viewed with suspicion the changes in clinical research, seeing in them a definition of clinical research close to that of the Nathan Committee. Some were deeply troubled by the way in which the *Roadmap* might pave the way for the pharmaceutical industry to exercise even greater influence over biomedical research and for the relationship between the NIH and the pharmaceutical industry. For Andrew Marks, Editor-in-Chief of the *Journal of Clinical Investigation,* the *Roadmap* was "not a road map at all, but a yellow brick road" and he was especially critical of any NIH involvement in large and hugely expensive clinical studies which he felt to be the responsibility of the pharmaceutical industry [42]. There was also concern that the thrust of the *Roadmap* lay in reductionist approaches that sought answer to health problems in molecular terms. Still others lamented that public health measures remained relatively neglected. In 2003, Claude Lenfant, Director of the National Heart Lung and Blood Institute in Bethesda, argued for more attention to "translation" in the last and, for him, the most important segment of the "translational highway" — medical practice at the community level [43].

The extent to which the NIH *Roadmap*, in establishing translational initiatives, influenced the development of translational initiatives beyond the United States remains an open question. During the 1990s, the HGP evolved into an international project, and its potential medical value was universally of interest. In the United Kingdom, where clinical research had from the 1990s been the subject of a number of reviews undertaken, for example, by the Department of Health and the Academy of Medical Sciences, the opening decade of the 21st century saw a number of reports urging the development of translational science/medicine/research as a means to "bridge" the "gap" between the lab and the clinic, between basic science and medicine, and also the "therapeutic gap" now seen to exist between the genome sequence and its clinical uses.[d] Several "translational" initiatives were launched, notably by the MRC in 2007, which established six Translational Medicine Centres ($15.5m/5 years) that, in the familiar "translational" rhetoric, would "enable scientific research to improve human health more quickly and efficiently," creating a new infrastructure to facilitate innovation.[e] Here too, close links with the pharmaceutical industry featured prominently. These centres would, it was hoped, "provide the pharmaceutical industry with a portal through which it can access the information it needs."[f]

The term "translation," variously applied to science, research, and/or medicine, was given form by the policies through which it was established as an approach to biomedical innovation in the

[d]Relevant policy reports in the United Kingdom include, for example: *Clinical Academic Careers*. (The Richards Report, 1997); *The tenure track clinician scientist: A new career pathway to promote recruitment into clinical practice* (Report of the Working Group on academic careers, March 2000); *Resuscitating clinical research in the UK* (Academy of Medical Sciences, 2002); *Strengthening clinical research*, Academy of Medical Sciences (2003); Cooksey, D. *A review of UK healthcare funding*, *HMSO*, London (2006).

[e]In 2004 in the United Kingdom, there were just 50 clinician-scientists, and an NHS R&D program created in 1994, which allocated 1.5% of total NHS expenditure to support clinical research, did not come to fruition.

[f]Professor Mike Hanna, UCL TM Centre. Cited in: Day, M., "MRC wants to cut time from bench to bedside", *BMJ* 334 (2007), p. 493.

21st century. Essentially, the term acts as a mechanism through which to effect change, changes prescribed in initiatives such as the NIH *Roadmap* and conceived of within senior biomedical policy circles. Its meaning is at once vague, because of the diverse activities, actors, and sectors involved in the process of biomedical innovation, but also highly specific, in that in practice it is defined differently by different actors (scientists, institutions, and so forth) in ways that reflect their position within the innovation process. As one pharmaceutical executive put it:

> Translation means different things to different people.... For pharma it is basically choosing the winners and dumping the losers. As a niche in academia, it is using the basic research and finding a home in early clinical to demonstrate that the thing works in man, as well as in yeast, or a mouse or a rat. And for the health care providers moving what seems to be an effective

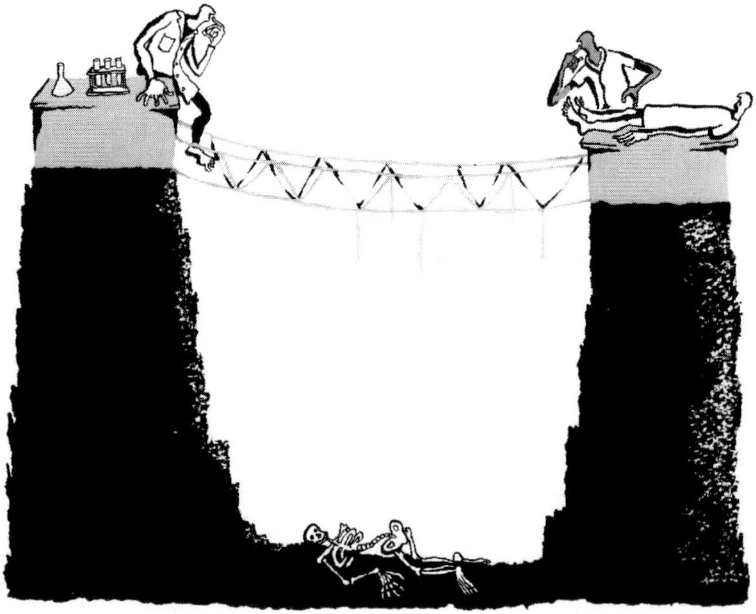

Figure 2.3 The "gap" between clinic and research laboratory: "Crossing the valley of death" (*Source*: Butler, D. [2008]. *Nature,* 453, pp. 840–842. Used with permission of Belle Mellor).

> therapy to actually change practice, and make a difference in terms of cost and benefit to how the NHS is run.[g]

The translational agenda remains in its infancy. In the United States, Elias Zerhouni resigned his post at the NIH ahead of the 2008 presidential election and it remains to be seen what will flow from the various initiatives established under the *Roadmap.* It is clear, however, that the seemingly intractable problems between the clinic and the lab persist. As late as 2008 the "gap" between them was depicted in an article in *Nature* as the "valley of death" (Fig. 2.3). Moreover, recent work by Dana Wilson-Kovacs and Christine Hauskeller confirms that the role of the clinician/physician-scientist in seeking to bridge the world of the clinic and the lab remains as troubled as ever [44].

2.4 Conclusion

This chapter has sought to show how the "translational turn" within contemporary biomedicine can be seen as a pragmatic response to long-standing problems in clinical research and between the clinic and the lab. It also proposes that the "translational turn" can be understood as a response to the HGP and the demands that the completion of this project would place on these parts of the biomedical enterprise. Into the 1960s in the United States, the physician-scientist formed an effective bridge between the clinic and the lab — "contradictory spheres of action." From this time onward, biomedical research was profoundly shaped by a seemingly irresistible commitment to molecular biology and its reductionist explanations of disease. With the growth of molecular biology, which both privileged the laboratory as the principal site for disease research and fostered specialization, the traditional dual role of the physician-scientist became unsustainable. Clinical research, especially the patient-centred kind, became unfashionable. For those building careers, the uncertainties and ambiguities inherent in this work — its "messiness" — was unattractive in comparison

[g]Interview with pharmaceutical executive, 4 June 2008.

with the highly and reliably productive world of the molecular biology laboratory. The shifting power relation between the lab and the clinic in the 1970s was undoubtedly influenced by the distribution of research funding, especially that of the all-powerful NIH. As Wyngaarden argued in 1979, resources flowed into the molecular biology laboratory to a much greater extent than was the case for patient-oriented clinical investigation. By the early 1990s, clinical research was considered by many — especially "embattled" physician-scientists — to be in crisis. These concerns went seemingly unnoticed, or at least without action, within senior biomedical policy circles. At the same time, the pharmaceutical industry — the major source of therapies for the biomedical enterprise — was also grappling with serious productivity and innovation problems. In the 1990s, key parts of the innovation chain were in difficulty.

Against this backdrop, work on the HGP continued apace. A great deal was riding on the HGP; it was imperative to reap the rewards — therapeutic, economic, scientific, and so forth — from the huge investment in this project. From its inception, the HGP proved transformative for the biomedical enterprise. This chapter has highlighted its influence on policy-making in relation to clinical research and at the lab-clinic interface during the 1990s. It has argued the significance of the HGP, even prior to its completion, in prompting renewed engagement with the long-standing, systemic problems in these "core" components of the biomedical enterprise. It charts the emergence within policy circles of a rhetoric which emphasized the need to reform clinical research in ways that would strengthen its relations with the laboratory in order to close the "gap" (or overcome "roadblocks") now seen to exist between these sites and which were now understood to be a serious impediment to innovation. This "gap" had intellectual, cultural, spatial, and temporal dimensions: all could be addressed by closer integration between the lab and the clinic which, so the reasoning went, would improve the efficiency of the innovation process. Such claims resonated strongly with the various constituencies with a "stake" in the HGP: the US government, the NIH, the pharmaceutical industry, the public, and the patient.

As the HGP approached completion, and in anticipation of this, policy-makers were forced to confront the serious problems within clinical research and between the clinic and the lab. The inertia of former times gave way to a new determination to address these problems, a determination fuelled by the need to realize in a timely manner the much-vaunted therapeutic potential of the HGP. The policy response took the form of the "translational turn." Endorsed at the highest levels in biomedical research and healthcare policy circles in the United States (and the United Kingdom), the emphasis on "translation" can be understood as a pragmatic response to long-standing problems in clinical research and at the interface between the clinic and the laboratory. The timing of this response reflected the imminent completion of the HGP and the demands that would follow in its wake. The "translational turn," initially apparent in policy discussions, has taken practical form in dedicated policy initiatives such as the NIH *Roadmap* (2003) and the MRC's Translational Medicine Centers (2006). It is within these initiatives that the term "translation" derives meaning. To its advocates, the rationale for the translational agenda lies in improving the pace of biomedical innovation to effect faster delivery of health benefits (especially, it might be argued, those deriving from the HGP) to the patient. Viewed this way, the "translational turn" appears necessary, desirable, and legitimate.

Others see it differently. Not everyone is enthralled with the "translational turn" — it has been, and remains contested, on a number of grounds. Critics argue that it works to seamlessly fold the HGP into the biomedical mission, casts the pharmaceutical industry in ever-closer partnership with state-funded actors, and establishes innovation as the explicit and primary goal of the biomedical "ecosystem." Elsewhere, there are reservations about its endorsement of the reductionism inherent in the HGP and reductionist approaches to the study of disease — which have flourished in the post-genomic era. Here, critics could point to the story of sickle cell anaemia (SCA) to bolster their argument. As noted, by the late 1950s the molecular basis of SCA had been resolved by Linus Pauling, Vernon Ingram, and others. However, effective treatments did not follow. Rather, the first effective therapy, hydroxyurea, was approved by the FDA only in 1998 — an advance which, as Valerie Williams has highlighted, arose in large part from clinical investigations involving physician-scientists [45]. This draws attention to fundamental differences between clinical and laboratory-based disease research: laboratory experiments act to simplify and control biological phenomena, whilst clinical investigations reflect to a greater degree the complexity, the "messiness" of the disease process in the whole patient. The SCA story points to the critical role that clinical investigation can play in developing effective therapies — a point long emphasized by physician-scientists. It is sobering to recall that, for all the insights, concepts, and techniques of molecular biology, and for all the investment in biomedical research — the cumulative budget of the NIH since 1950 stands at over $400bn — prevalent diseases, such as cancer and heart disease, remain largely incurable. Whether in the wake of the "translational turn" this situation can be improved upon remains to be seen.

References

1. Wainwright, S.P., Cribb, A., Michael, M., and Williams, C. (2009). Stem cells, translational research and the sociology of science, in: Atkinson, P. Glasner, P., and Lock, M. (eds) *Handbook of Genetics & Society: Mapping the New Genomic Era*. Routledge, London.
2. Maulitz, R.C. (1979). Physician versus bacteriologist: The ideology of science in clinical medicine. In: Vogel, M.V., and Rosenberg, C. (eds) *The Therapeutic Revolution. Essays on the Social History of American Medicine.* University of Pennsylvania Press, Philadelphia. pp. 91–107.
3. Lowy, I. (1987). The impact of medical practice on biomedical research: The case of human leucocyte antigens studies, *Minerva,* **25**, pp. 171–200.
4. Culliton, B. (1995). Clinical investigation: An endangered science, *Nature Medicine,* **1**, p. 281.
5. Topping, N.H. (1952). The US Public Health Service Clinical Center for Medical Research, *Journal of the American Medical Association*, **150**, pp. 541–545.

6. Landsborough Thomson, A. (1975). *Half a Century of Medical Research.* (Volume II). HMSO, London.
7. Faber, K. (1930). *Nosography: The Evolution of Clinical Medicine in Modern Times. (2nd Ed).* Hoeber, New York.
8. Shear, M.J. (1951). Role of the chemotherapy research laboratory in clinical cancer research, *Journal of the National Cancer Institute*, **12,** pp. 569–581.
9. Rosenberg, L.E. (1999). The physician-scientist: An essential – and fragile – link in the medical research chain, *Journal of Clinical Investigation*, **103**, pp. 1621–1626.
10. Seldin, D.W. (1966). Some reflections on the role of basic research and service in clinical departments, *Journal of Clinical Investigation,* **45**(6), pp. 976–979.
11. Fox Keller, E. (1990). Physics and the emergence of molecular biology: A history of cognitive and political synergy, *Journal of the History of Biology,* **23**(3), pp. 389–409.
12. Kay, Lily E. (1993). *The Molecular Vision of Life.* Oxford University Press, Oxford.
13. Strasser, B. (2002). Institutionalizing molecular biology in post-war Europe: A comparative study, *Studies in the History and Philosophy of the Biological and Biomedical Sciences,* **33**, pp. 533–564.
14. Pauling, L., Itano, H.A., Singer, S.J., and Wells, I.C. (1949). Sickle cell anemia, a Molecular Disease, *Science* **110**, pp. 543–548.
15. Strasser, B. (1999). Sickle cell anemia, a Molecular Disease, *Science,* **286**(5444), pp. 1488–1490.
16. Fox Keller, E. (1992). Nature versus nurture, in: Kevles, D., and Hood, L. *Code of Codes* Harvard University Press, Boston MA.
17. De Chadarevian, S. (2002). *Designs for Life. Molecular Biology after World War II.* Cambridge University Press, Cambridge.
18. Keating, P., and Cambrosio, A. (2004). Does biomedicine entail the successful reduction of pathology to biology?, *Perspectives in Biology and Medicine,* **47**(3), pp. 357–371.
19. Nathan, D.G. (1998). *Clinical Research.* Perceptions, reality and proposed solutions, *Journal of the American Medical Association,* **280**, pp. 1427–1431.
20. Wyngaarden, J.B. (1979). The clinical investigator as an endangered species, *New England Journal of Medicine,* **301**, pp. 1254–1259.
21. Gill, G.N. (1984). The end of the physician-scientist, *American Scholar,* **53**, pp. 353–368.

22. Kubinyi, H. (2003). Drug research: Myths, hype and reality, *Nature Reviews Drug Discovery,* **2**, pp. 665–668.

23. Thompson, J.N., and Moskowitz, J. (1997). Preventing the extinction of the clinical research ecosystem, *Journal of the American Medical Association*, **278,** pp. 241–245.

24. Ahrens, E.H. (1992). *The Crisis in Clinical Research. Overcoming Institutional Obstacles.* Oxford University Press, Oxford.

25. Goldstein, J.L., and Brown, M.S. (1997). The clinical investigator: Bewitched, bothered and bewildered – but still beloved, *Journal of Clinical Investigation,* **99**(12), pp. 2803–2812.

26. Kelley, W.N., and Randolph, M.A. (eds) (1994). *Careers in clinical research: Obstacles and Opportunities.* National Academy Press, Washington, D.C.

27. NIH Director's Panel on Clinical Research Report, December 1997. http://www.nih.gov/news/crp/97report/index.htm.

28. For a rejection of the Nathan Committee definition of clinical research, see: Schechter, A. (1998). The crisis in clinical research. Endangering the half century NIH consensus, *Journal of the American Medical Association,* **280**, pp. 1440–1442.

29. Rees, J. (2002). Complex disease and the new clinical sciences, *Science,* **296**, pp. 698–700.

30. Sung, N.S., Crowley, W.F., Genel, M. *et al.* (2003). Central challenges facing the national clinical research enterprise, *Journal of the American Medical Association*, **289,** pp. 1278–1287.

31. Vos, R. (1991). *Drugs Looking for Diseases: Innovative Drug Research and the Development of the Beta Blockers and the Calcium Antagonists.* Kluwer Academic, Dordrecht.

32. Wright, S. (1986). Recombinant DNA technology and it social transformation, *Osiris*, **2**, pp. 303–360.

33. Smith Hughes, S. (2001). Making dollars out of DNA: The first major patent in biotechnology and the commercialization of molecular biology, 1974–1980, *Isis,* **92**, pp. 541–575.

34. Kleinman, D.L. (2005). *Science and Technology in Society: From Biotechnology to the Internet.* Oxford University Press, Oxford.

35. Bell, J. (2005). Resuscitating clinical research in the UK, *British Medical Journal,* **327,** pp. 1041–1043.

36. Kevles, D.J. (1997). Big science and big politics in the US: Reflections on the death of the super conducting super collider and the life of the

human genome project, *Historical Studies in the Physical and Biological Sciences*, **27**, pp. 269–298.

37. Watson, J.D. (1990). The human genome project: Past, present and future, *Science*, **248**, pp. 44–51.
38. Kraft, A., and Rothman, H. (2008). Genomics-based drug innovation: Visions and commercial viability, *International Journal of Biotechnology*, **10**(5), pp. 441–460.
39. Zerhouni, E. (2003). The NIH roadmap, *Science*, **302**, pp. 63–72.
40. Zerhouni, E. A., and Alving, B. (2006). *Translational Research*, **148**, pp. 4–5.
41. Weissman, G. (2005). Roadmaps, translational research and childish curiosity, *FASEB Journal*, **19**, pp. 1761–1762.
42. Marks, A.R. (2006). Rescuing the NIH before it is too late, *Journal of Clinical Investigation*, **116(**4), p. 844.
43. Lenfant, C. (2003). Clinical research to clinical practice — lost in translation?, *New England Journal of Medicine*, **349**, pp. 868–874.
44. Wilson-Kovacs, D., and Hauskeller, C. (2012) The clinician-scientist: Professional dynamics in clinical stem cell research, *Sociology of Health and Illness*, **34**(4), pp. 497–512.
45. Williams, V.L. (2004). Pathways of innovation. A history of the first effective treatment for sickle cell anemia, *Perspectives in Biology and Medicine*, **47**(4), pp. 552–563.

Chapter 3

Translational Medicine: The Industry Perspective

Christopher-Paul Milne[a,*] **and Christine Kohn**[b]

[a]*Center for the Study of Drug Development, Tufts University Medical School, 75 Kneeland St., Suite 1100, Boston, MA 02111, USA*

[b]*University of Connecticut/Hartford Hospital Evidence-Based Practice Center, Hartford Hospital, 80 Seymour Street, Hartford, CT 06102-5037, USA*

*christopher.milne@tufts.edu

3.1 Introduction

Why are pharmaceutical companies embracing translational medicine (TM)? The answer is mainly because it is practical; they must increase productivity and remain competitive. Drug developers seeking to improve R&D productivity are pursuing extrinsic strategies, which include mergers and acquisitions, partnerships, and licensing. At the same time they are looking to implement intrinsic strategies, such as deciding which disease areas to pursue through portfolio optimization, integration of tools, technologies, approaches to development, and selection of appropriate milestones. Companies need to make better decisions about what

Translational Medicine: The Future of Therapy
Edited by James Mittra and Christopher-Paul Milne

ISBN 978-981-4316-99-6 (Hardback), 978-981-4364-84-3 (eBook)
www.panstanford.com

targets to pursue, when and how to terminate specific development programs, how to efficiently allocate resources, and what type of development portfolio to build. Although many traditional drug development approaches still have utility, they likely won't produce drug candidates at the pace the industry needs [1]. For one thing, the medical information and research literature is so diverse, sometimes contradictory, and becomes obsolete so fast that using it to assess the commercial prospects of a medical product are generally confusing, sometimes erroneous, and potentially dangerous. Translational science, especially in medicine, is providing a better way to identify promising molecules earlier in drug development by establishing the drug's risk/benefit profile earlier, for example, through the use of biomarkers or better animal-to-human models [2]. In recent years, all major pharmaceutical companies have implemented TM activities in tandem with their traditional drug discovery and development schemes. The mission of this new entity, which is different from TM as an academic discipline, is simply to improve predictability of the potential success of compounds as they transit through the different stages of drug development toward fulfilling a medical benefit [3]. While the mission of TM for industry is more intensely and narrowly focused than it is for academia, industry is motivated by much the same drivers and uses the same basic tools as the academic discipline.

The information sources and inspiration for this chapter derive from the affiliation of one its authors (CPM) with the Center for the Study of Drug Development (CSDD) at the Tufts University Medical School (TUSM). TUSM is one of several score academic institutions funded through the NIH's Clinical Translational Science Awards to advance the application of basic science research to human medical treatments. CSDD's role has been to explore the role the biopharmaceutical industry can play in furthering those efforts. Some of the data and case studies discussed in this chapter emerged from the academic–industry panels and workshops which have been held to explore the benefits and logistics of such private–public collaborations.

3.2 Translational Medicine Drivers

3.2.1 *Patient-Centered Approach*

In the past, new drugs were developed independently of the clinic, and often then "thrown over the fence" for safety testing in clinical trials, but now the fences are being pulled down to facilitate the back-and-forth movement in the "bench-to-bedside" feedback loop [2]. In concert with the momentum in the public sector, many major pharmaceutical firms in the private sector have formed TM units, whose goal in the broadest sense is to create a more direct connection between basic research and patient care. As the head of oncology at the international pharmaceutical company AstraZeneca put it, "We want to address the question of how our drugs actually work in man" [4]. This aim is being pursued by conducting first-in-human studies (FIH) earlier in the development process of a promising compound, by using healthy volunteers instead of patients to test efficacy through experiments rather than time and resource-consuming clinical trials. For example, there is an experimental medicine TM consortium working on, among other projects, an anxiety challenge study. In this study, anxiety is first artificially created in volunteers with a pharmacological agent in a laboratory setting and then the responses of the volunteers to a putative therapeutic agent are analyzed. Another approach associated with the expedited use of new drugs in human volunteers is the use of microdoses, so-called phase 0 studies conducted in volunteers with pharmacologically inactive doses that can still provide important early clues on toxicity and pharmacokinetics. This is considered to be acceptable on an ethical basis because the doses are so minute as to be similar to the amount of foreign substances that we are exposed to everyday from the environment [4].

In a patient-centered approach to clinical trials, there is an increased emphasis on early patient testing and evaluation on the part of bench researchers (jumping the T1 gap from basic science to human application) but also a more data-driven approach on the part of the medical practitioners in the clinic (jumping the T2 gap from human application to actual clinical utility and providing a nexus with the evidence-based medicine movement). In a TM approach, for instance when a new drug is first being considered, instead of asking how big the market is, it would ask: What and how great will be the variations in individual responses both in terms of efficacy and safety; and can we classify them on the basis of biomarkers that are either available or conceptually possible? Furthermore, in a TM approach outcomes data are sought up front, not as an afterthought for product lifecycle management. Patient views and feelings regarding side effects, treatment response, and QOL are increasingly important to the comparative effectiveness of the drug. Many companies are gathering data through surveys and patient diaries, typically by remote monitoring through telemetry or electronic communications. TM's patient-centered approach also extends to expanding options for assessing the prognosis of a disease and its treatment, as well as the use of diagnostics that are non-invasive and minimize patient discomfort [2].

For example, positron emission tomography (PET) and single-photon emission computed tomography (SPECT), which measure indirect markers of electrical activity in the brain, and EEG (electroencephalography) which measure this directly, are neuroimaging techniques to confirm that a molecule has crossed the blood brain barrier (BBB) and reached its site of action. However, new studies have shown promise for an even more convenient and efficient way to track functional brain activity in clinical drug development trials — magnetoencephalography (MEG). From a patient prospective, MEG is easier to set up and use in a consistent manner and is non-invasive and safe. From a provider prospective, it has shown a superior ability to measure brain activity and has seen routine use in certain areas of neurosurgery. From a drug development perspective, recent work illustrates its utility for central nervous system (CNS) pharmacodynamics. Similarly, specific anomalies in the MEG signatures are able to characterize a wide range of neurological diseases and conditions such as Alzheimer's disease, Schizophrenia, Parkinson's disease, pain, depression, and tinnitus. Pharma companies have found that the best data are generated from the integration of both current and breakthrough neuroimaging as complementary technologies. Making clinical trials more efficient and less burdensome to patients allows companies to target larger patient populations with less cost, and yield more generalizable results, thus improving prospects for better lifecycle management of the drug for both regulatory and commercial purposes [1].

3.2.2 *Payers*

Payers, frustrated with the lack of effectiveness for many products for many diseases with high healthcare costs (see Fig. 3.1), are also driving the adoption of TM concepts. Philosophically, they favor an approach called the Medical Home concept, which focuses on the whole person rather than a single disease or organ. The emphasis is on personalized care and decision-making by patients in partnership with their physicians. On the practical side, payers are requiring more and more comparative–effectiveness research (CER) and patient-reported outcomes (PRO) data on new and standard treatments, which has led to the rise of patient registries. Patient registries are databases containing information on patients with specific conditions, and have several advantages over randomized clinical trials (RCTs). First, they can follow patients over a longer period of time than RCTs. Second, they better reflect the management of a condition in its particular health microenvironment. Third, they evolve over time, along with new data and changing influences on clinical practice. Fourth, they bring into focus the impact of co-morbidities and concomitant treatments on patient outcomes. Finally, they can be effectively linked to electronic health records, patient questionnaires, and other complementary data. Also, patient registries have much less susceptibility to the usual factors limiting the scope of patient studies, such as time, geography, size of the sample, and participating health care providers. For example, the REACH registry for atherothrombosis encompassed over 60,000 patients and 4 years of follow-up, included patients in 44 countries, and involved close to 5,000 health care providers [4]. Although patient registries were in use before the TM current reached mainstream R&D, they have become much more common within a patient-centered research environment, increasing by 20% year-over-year since the early 2000s [5]. With its emphasis on PROs and documenting relative effectiveness in real-world settings, patient registries complement the bench-to-bedside loop as well as

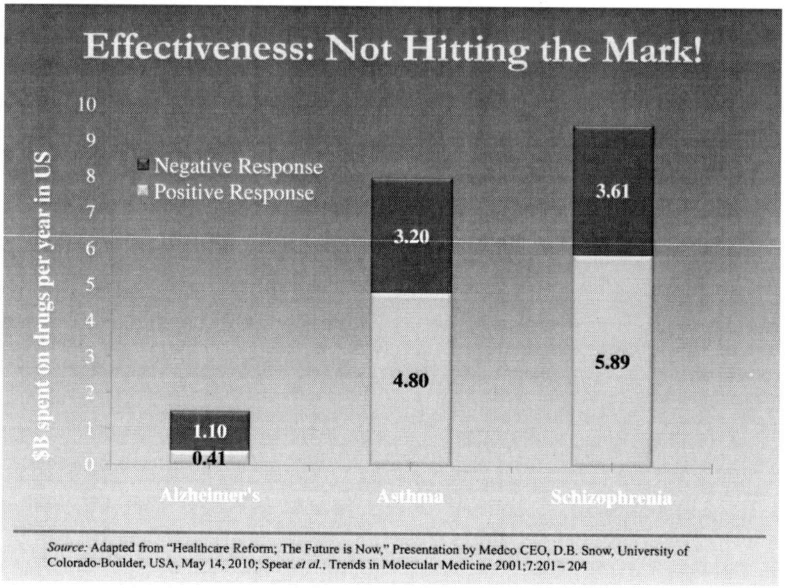

Figure 3.1 Health spending for drugs that lack effectiveness.

help to establish the value proposition that may make drugs more competitive at gaining good formulary placement from third-party payers.

TM can be used by companies to explore competitive advantage for market placement. For example, one company is looking at a GLP-1 agonist for the treatment of type 2 diabetes mellitus, which, based on its mechanism of action would be a direct competitor for Byetta (generic, exenatide, marketed by Amylin and Eli Lilly). Byetta has a dose-limiting side effect of nausea and vomiting, while pre-clinical data for the study drug suggests that it is well tolerated, having a better therapeutic window and a lower incidence of side effects. By taking data from the test drug's tolerability and PK/PD studies, as well as data from Byetta, study designs and decision trees based on the possible outcomes of each trial for the test drug have been formulated. Using an active comparator arm in clinical trials allows for the direct comparison of the trial drug with the current standard of therapy (in this case, Byetta). This TM approach can demonstrate early on if the new medication has a place in therapy and on the market, and whether payers will pay, patients will have a better therapeutic option, and whether the company should continue to invest or re-direct their resources [1].

3.2.3 *Education*

The divide between basic and applied research is a no man's land where on the one side there are molecular biologists who think simply in cellular terms and on the other side are clinicians who are more physiologically oriented. What is actually required is a good mix of people who can meet in the middle, but many in the highly specialized world of R&D are not equipped to think translationally, creating the need for researchers and clinicians who are both more academic and science oriented [6]. TM programs are being implemented to jump the gap by creating a common language for effective and productive communication among the various stakeholders, and by encouraging programs within the different institutions to foster the exchange of technologies and ideas. A good example at the level of individual companies is Serono's use of "back translation" by researchers to enhance clinicians' understanding of complex disease processes, such as defective remyelination in MS, so they can use their feedback to do trials in animals that mirror what might be done in man [7].

At a more macro level, the perception of a budding job market for translationists has led to the creation of a host of new training and degree programs at academic centers to teach a new cadre of clinicians and researchers how to think beyond the traditional — and outdated — boundaries of institutional scope, and to focus on one of the ultimate goals of basic research: improving health care by bringing newer and better treatments to the patient [4]. Many universities have had MD-PhD programs for a number of years to help create a cadre of physician researchers. Now there are also several innovative programs, which are much shorter, and can benefit both academic and industry scientists such as 1-year certificates in clinical and translational sciences or Masters of Medical Programs for science PhDs. In addition, there are ways for those on what has traditionally been a long slog through MD or PhD programs to "see how the other half lives" through a "one-year out" program encompassing a year outside the medical school to conduct research and development, or the "Med into Grad" program, in which PhD students take 1.5 years of medical school alongside the medical students (>dozen such programs have been launched by the Howard Hughes Medical Institute (HHMI) and Doris Dukes Foundation [7].

3.2.4 *Industry–Academic Collaboration*

Another stratagem adopted by industry to improve productivity is both extrinsic and intrinsic in nature. Companies must realign themselves organizationally to eliminate research silos that have kept industry R&D insulated from innovative thinking within and without its own walls. Drug developers are increasingly forming partnerships with universities and research hospitals to identify breakthroughs in basic research that may translate into clinical development opportunities. On the industry side, motivation in this case is not only the weak pipeline for new products, but also the need to access more talent and fresh ideas. On the academic side, stagnant funding from public sector sources (i.e., the budget of the US National Institutes of Health has flatlined in recent years), increasing competition for faculty, and the ability to attract top-tier students make industry collaboration appealing [1]. Motivating both sides is the desire to access the raw materials of R&D; namely biological samples. On the one hand, large numbers of blood samples exist, particularly among CROs that have conducted clinical trials for drug company clients, and could provide a treasure trove for academic researchers. Accessing those data is problematic, however, since the patients who donated their blood often did not give their consent for use of those samples for medical research, but partnering programs may provide an avenue to avoid pro forma barriers [1]. On the other hand, academic medical centers (AMC), operating under the auspices of major universities, have access to large patient populations, and have the facilities to manage high-risk patients as well as an interest in areas of high unmet medical needs. A recent review by Tufts University Medical School of over 3,000 industry–academic collaborations at medical schools in 15 states demonstrates an array of programs that address a number of needs in TM (see Table 3.1). While the majority of those collaborations

Table 3.1 Sample subset of industry–AMC collaborations in TM

TM categories	Number of projects	Example
Bio-imaging	10	MRI identification of hi-risk patients with RA
Animal models	9	Transgenic mouse model for Alzheimer's disease
Biomarkers	8	Systemic genotoxicity bio- marker for IBD inflammation
Training & education	4	Imaging training set for future radiopharmaceuticals in PD
T2/T3	4	Care coordination in small facility, CV/diabetes patients
Breakthrough technology	2	Green Light Hi-Performance System for treating BPH
Master agreements	2	"MA translational research": East Carolina U. & Merck/SP
Bioinformatics	1	2-hydroxyglutarate metabolism signatures/ glioma

were clinical trials focused on specific products, over 10% were special programs that had a broader focus or impact on biomedical R&D. Within the sub-group of special programs were 40 that could be described as translational.

Some of the examples illustrate cross-over areas where TM goals for both industry and academia are closely aligned and capacities are synergistic. For example, with regard to animal models, basic research in academia was very good at uncovering the workings of biological pathways, just not necessarily human ones. There were problems in bridging the gaps between results from *in vitro, in vivo,* and *in silico* experiments. Animal models were often not predictive enough for human disease (famously demonstrated recently in the TGN 1412 trial in which six human volunteers suffered multiple-organ failure despite the fact that monkeys had been administered a dose 500 times higher without apparent ill effect), or were practically nonexistent for some biotechnology approaches (for example, monoclonal antibodies that target human proteins often have specific effects in humans that are not conducive to animal testing). Thinking began to change when the

Human Genome Project, which focused the attention of clinicians on molecular biology, opened up the possibilities of personalized medicine and refocused science on the human laboratory, a clarion call heard by the proponents of TM [4]. In similar vein, the University of Connecticut/Sanofi program to track patients with type 2 diabetes and heart disease at small primary care centers for 12 months — utilizing electronic health record systems (EHRS) to coordinate care with the goal of narrowing the gap between theory and practice in care coordination — is at the heart of the TM goal to bring innovations to community-based clinics, rural or otherwise. Likewise, the University of Arizona/Alseres effort to collect data to populate an imaging training set for future trials of diagnostically uncertain tremor in Parkinson's disease, even though such radiopharmaceuticals remain unapproved by FDA, addresses the TM goal to anticipate training needs for medical innovations and facilitate their uptake in clinical practice.

3.3 Biomarkers, Bioimaging, Bioinformatics: Industrial Strength TM Tools

The conceptual impetus for TM within industry was likely a by-product of the adoption of Model-Based Drug Development (MBDD), derived from the yet earlier learn–confirm strategy for drug development emerging in the 1990s. In MBDD, drug development is viewed as a continuous process during which new data are acquired as animal and human studies are conducted. It should be emphasized that MBDD starts before a compound is selected for preclinical development by defining the PK-PD strategy, biomarkers, and animal studies that will support translation to humans. The data from each new clinical study must be integrated with relevant previous information to inform decision-making (e.g., design the next study or terminate the development of the new compound). A common limitation of the current drug development strategy is that prior information is partly or completely ignored when analyzing and interpreting the results of the most recent clinical trial. Models allow us to integrate data from different studies in a logical manner based on our understanding of the drug and disease. Thus, under an

MBDD approach drug development is viewed as a model building exercise during which we continuously translate our knowledge about a new compound and use this knowledge to inform our decision-making and drug development strategy [8].

An MBDD approach explains a shift toward science-based development where study and modeling data are integrated logically and based on understanding disease pathology and drug parameters to inform decision-making in the next immediate step (i.e., should the study proceed as planned, be redesigned, or should further development be stopped). Utilized properly, it carries wide potential to look at the entire scope of data and address inadequacies that have become inherent in the process. It informs go/no-go decisions and builds understanding of compound behavior through the integration of data across the discovery–development spectrum. It allows for the analysis of assumptions through trial simulation by exploring the impact of variables, such as dose selection, patient population, and trial design, while simultaneously integrating all available knowledge. In so doing, companies can often avoid investing in studies that will likely fail or elicit unusable or unneeded data. Quantitatively informing trial design and picking a dose based on methodologies that are based on actual data increases the likelihood of success in both clinical trials and with regulatory affairs. Benchmarking against competitors keeps a product from being developed in a vacuum and ensures it will have a place on the market. The capacity to make go/no-go decisions in early development by incorporating advanced biomarkers and other predictive tools (for example, those employing bioinformatics and bioimaging) in Phase I and early Phase II studies allows for the demonstration of proof-of-concept earlier in the process and more accurately. In that way quicker and smarter decisions can be made to pursue compounds or reinvest resources into more promising opportunities [6].

3.3.1 *Biomarkers*

The development and refinement of biomarkers was identified by the FDA in the United States and EMA in Europe as a key effort in the medical product development process to improve knowledge and efficiency. In Europe, this effort has been initiated through collaboration with the Innovation Think Tank of the EMA Committee for Medicinal Products for Human Use (EMA/CHMP) to support a TM approach for R&D of safety/efficacy biomarkers. While in the United States, several implicit TM initiatives were launched in response to the call-to-arms for research on biomarkers and advanced disease modeling published in the FDA's Critical Path Initiative (CPI) document [7]. One of the most ambitious of these initiatives has been the Biomarker Consortium, which is a collaboration of approximately 40 companies, not-for-profits, advocacy groups, and government to develop and qualify biomarkers for cancer, metabolic, neuropsychiatric, inflammatory, and autoimmune disorders. One of the most active of these initiatives has been the Predictive Safety Testing Consortium (PSTC), whose members include scientists from global pharmaceutical companies, academia, and government. The PSTC was organized and is led by the Critical Path Institute (C-Path), a not-for-profit organization that works to facilitate FDA participation in research collaborations. In 2008, the FDA and the EMA approved seven key proteins, or biomarkers, found in urine that can provide additional information regarding drug-induced damage to kidney cells, also known as renal toxicity. This advance was made possible by a new regulatory communication process implemented by the PSTC, which enabled it not only to submit a single biomarker data application to both regulatory agencies, but also to meet jointly with scientists from both agencies to discuss it in detail and address scientific questions posed by the regulators [7].

Within industry, there are thousands of biomarkers being used at various stages of R&D and are an integral part of the translational jump from late discovery to early clinical development (see Fig. 3.2). In fact, it was suggested at a recent industry panel meeting [1] that a biomarker plan outlining target engagement, pharmacodynamic assays, proof of biology, and proof of concept should be developed 1–2 years before lead optimization for each potential developmental candidate. Periodic ongoing reviews of the progress in biomarker development should be required, and tracked as if it were a product in development with cross-functional input and prioritization of efforts and funding toward biomarker discovery, validation, and clinical qualification [1].

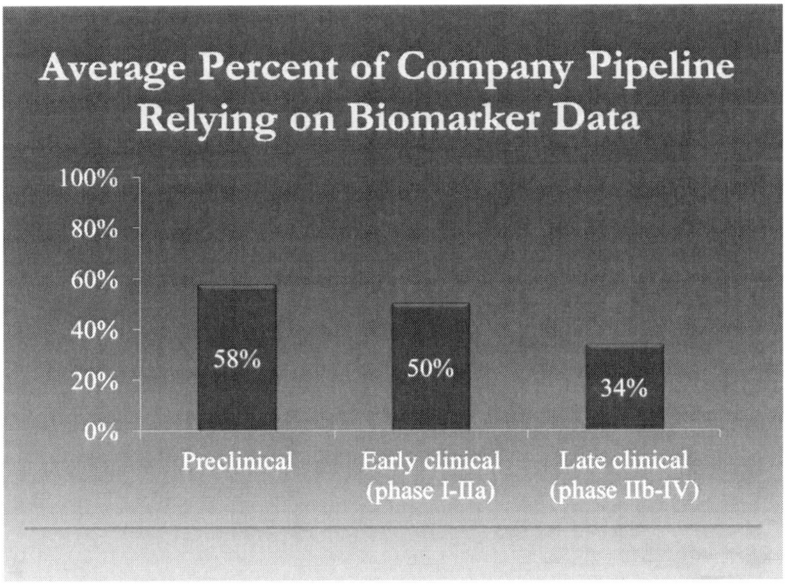

Figure 3.2 Use of biomarkers increasing in products earlier in pipeline.

Biomarkers have emerged as a trademark tool of TM and form the basis for promising commercial applications in personalized medicine. To overcome the scientific and resource challenges of drug-diagnostic development, there is an especially compelling incentive for companies to partner in this field. Abbott recently received approval from the FDA for a new molecular diagnostic test designed to detect rearrangements of the anaplastic lymphoma kinase (ALK) gene in non-small-cell lung cancer (NSCLC). Importantly, the new test was designed as a companion diagnostic to identify ALK-positive patients for Pfizer's newly approved NSCLC therapy, an oral first-in-class ALK inhibitor [6]. Still, from an industry perspective, biomarkers are very much a work in progress. On the one hand, they are proving enormously valuable in the development of personalized medicines, while on the other hand, two major challenges need to be overcome before they will be fully embraced by drug developers. First, the economics of patient recruitment for diseases that affect relatively small numbers of patients are very challenging. For example, to attract 500 patients with a designated genotype in a disease area with 4% prevalence requires screening 12,500 patients. That number jumps to 17,500 when one accounts for likely patient dropout during trials. Second, developers commonly use biomarkers to better understand patient response, but have rarely relied on them when seeking regulatory approval, because few regulatory standards for acceptable biomarkers have been established [1]. Nonetheless, biomarkers may serve to streamline R&D dramatically, shaving off perhaps as much as $100m and 3–4 years from the resources currently expended for the R&D of a novel medicine [6].

3.3.2 *Bioimaging*

As important as biomarkers themselves are, imaging biomarkers and accompanying technology are on a very short list of new TM tools with the most immediate impact. For example, of the top 30 most highly rated medical innovations, nine were biomarkers, and of these, four were imaging biomarkers [9]. The EMA supports the view that they have an important role to play, and believes that new imaging techniques and end points build confidence in biological rationale, and are more sensitive than clinical end points, especially for disease-modifying products. The FDA adds that C-Path will concentrate on imaging biomarkers because of their particular utility for distinguishing biologically based subsets for neuropsychiatric diseases, and through its Molecular Assay and Targeted Therapeutics (MATT) project is undertaking integrated development of drugs, diagnostics and imaging technology for cancer care. At the same time, the multi-company Biomarker Consortium is working on imaging standardization methods, approved proposals for a MRI study to measure and differentiate plaque, and positron emission tomography (PET) biomarkers for diagnosing brain disorders [7].

Among the advantages that imaging offers are the availability of imaging endpoints associated with disease phenotypes, its ability to provide a dynamic view of disease and bioactivity of a drug, and the fact that imaging is species-independent and fully translational. Already used in clinical settings, imaging offers the prospect of smaller, less expensive, and more efficient pre-clinical studies.

Intravital microscopy enables researchers to look inside living cells, making it possible to image cell-specific distribution and effects of drugs in organs of living animals [1].

As with the R&D of genetic biomarkers for companion diagnostics, the incentive to collaborate on bioimaging projects is very compelling because of the variety of technologies and the vastness of the expertise required rarely resides in one company, even if they are major biopharmaceutical companies with thousands of scientists and billion dollar R&D budgets. Recently, for example, J&J and Pfizer have been working collaboratively on specialized imaging biomarkers to track the effect of a candidate monoclonal antibody on Alzheimer's patient burden of beta-amyloid in the brain [6]. We will illustrate this further by discussing a case study (see next section) of the Alzheimer's Disease Neuroimaging Initiative (ADNI), an ambitious multi-year, multi-company collaboration, begun in 2004, to study changes of cognition, function, brain structure and function, and biomarkers in elderly subjects with mild cognitive impairment, and those with Alzheimer's disease (AD).

3.3.3 *Bioinformatics*

Bioinformatics manages and decodes "omic" data and facilitates the TM concept by helping to distribute such information throughout the entire healthcare value chain. Beyond the basic goals of compiling, accessing, and organizing data in a comprehensible and transferable manner, TM seeks the higher goal of maximizing the use of data. Programs such as CPI's Clinical Data Interchange Standards Consortium, which has approximately 300 corporate sponsors, are taking on the challenging task of standardizing and managing data in order to produce generalized knowledge from the vast amounts of raw data being generated. Bioinformatics covers a variety of activities: sequence assembly (computer-based assembly of fragments); genomic sequence analysis (gene-mapping); functional genomics; genotyping (identifying individual disease susceptibility); proteomics (e.g., microarrays); pharmacogenomics (e.g., SNP databases); and database administration (maintenance of huge databases of genomic sequence and biochemical information and development of intelligent search algorithms).

Genetic and biochemical information companies are focused on developing high-throughput technologies such as next-generation DNA sequencing; multiplex assays; microarray-based and chip-based genotyping and proteomic profiling tools; and metabolic tools that better assess S&E to answer up front questions that used to take weeks, sometimes in a matter of minutes. For example, Caliper Life Sciences recently launched a microfluidics platform that allows companies to conduct precise high-throughput tests on DNA and RNA samples 70 times faster than conventional methods [6].

The effective management of knowledge in translational research setting is a major challenge and opportunity for pharmaceutical research and development companies. The wealth of data generated in experimental medicine studies and clinical trials can inform the quest for next generation drugs, but only if all the data generated during those studies are appropriately collected, managed, and shared. Some notable successes have already been achieved. Merck has developed a system which enables sharing of human subject data in oncology trials with the Moffit Cancer Center and Research Institute. There is a growing set of functional genomics data being deposited in a variety of publicly accessible databases such as the US National Center for Biotechnology Information (NCBI) GEO, European Bioinformatics Institute (EBI) Array Express, Stanford Microarray Database, and the caGRID infrastructure, which is derived from gene expression experiments on tissue samples collected from clinical settings. Many of those are from either drug discovery or biomarker discovery projects. In particular, Johnson & Johnson through its subsidiaries has contributed such data sets into GEO and Array Express [10].

An important nexus for translational medicine and bioinformatics is facilitating the integration of information from biobanks, which store biological samples of hundreds or thousands of patients with the associated characteristics (genetic information, collection conditions, medical history, etc). The appropriate association and interpretation of this information reveal the key biomarkers for early detection of diseases [11]. The treasure trove of high-content data derived from human samples can be much more effectively mined if standard dictionaries applied to all these studies and each subject's clinical record and the associated sample's genomics data is stored and analyzed through a system which enables efficient access and mining [10].

3.4 Case Studies

3.4.1 *Translational Neuroscience Efforts*

CNS drug development has stalled for a plethora of reasons, including issues with pharmacologic target identification, a lag in the turnover of neurobiology research to the CNS drug development process, and insufficient technologies to help identify lead compounds that may have significant value in treating CNS disorders. For example, in cardiovascular disease, there are biomarkers such as blood pressure and cholesterol levels that help to track cardiovascular health, disease progression, and treatment goals. In contrast, even the most fundamental CNS functions, such as cognitive testing, lack standardization, and global acceptance in clinical practice. The lack of such standards not only affects diagnosis, but also patient management. Such differences have made CNS drug development a long and expensive endeavor with uncertain success.

Pharmaceutical companies are seeking progressive technologies for the study of neurophysiology with the specific application of adapting them in the development of personalized CNS medicines. Advances in computers and telecommunication technologies offer the possibility of bringing routine, objective CNS (central nervous system) measures into mainstream health care, and could build on cutting edge technologies already in use in early drug development for collecting neurophysiological data. Early translational research efforts to this effect have looked to the advances in computers and telecommunication in order to bring routine, objective CNS tests into conventional practice. Indeed, several commercial technologies may show promise in developing and measuring personalized CNS biomarkers that are patient-friendly. Cell phones and computers may allow for the tracking of baseline behaviors which could then be used as a comparator to quantitatively track changes in clinical endpoints, such as cognitive function, disease progression, and treatment response. Certain pharma companies hope that this

Table 3.2 New technologies and scientific/business collaborations to advance personalized medicines mentioned by Tufts CSDD study respondents

New technologies already incorporated or planning to use in personalized medicine development programs	Collaborations or private–public partnerships to advance personalized medicine (number of respondents participating is given in parentheses)
Genomics, proteomics, metabolomics	Personalized Medicine Coalition (5×)
Transcriptome, RNAi	Critical Path (USA) and/or Innovative Medicines Initiative (EU) (4×)
DME characterization, expanded and earlier use of biomarkers	The Biomarkers Consortium (3×)
DNA/Next Gen sequencing, SNiPs	Industry PGx Working Group (2×)
Biosimulations, animal models coupled w/*in vitro* patient samples	International SAE Consortium (2×)
Phenomics, informational genomics	TM Alliance (aka Kauffman Foundation) (2×)
Integration Analytical Modeling	TI Pharma (the Netherlands-based P-P-P)
Circulating Tumor Cells (CTC)	Oncology Biomarker Program
Tumor Gene Signatures	Hi-Risk Imaging Group
"Smart" Reagents for bio-imaging, neuro-imaging compounds	Karolinska Institute
Histochemistry, phase 0, gene therapy	Anti-TNF rheumatoid arthritis Consortium

could lead to a new generation of novel, objective, and personalized behavioral biomarkers. Single lead, dry EEG electrodes have already been incorporated into personalized sleep monitoring systems which are sent, via the Internet, so sleep patterns can be monitored. It is the ability to validate, standardize, and then incorporate their use in drug development and disease management that will increase efficiency and output of the development process. More research needs to be conducted to determine if these technologies can be used to determine specific brain biomarkers and to track disease progression and medication safety and efficacy. If this is accomplished and regulatory bodies also adopt these new industry standards, the operation of clinical trials and drug development as a whole could be transformed. Studies could be performed remotely with little burden on patient volunteers. Translational research has the broad perspective and foresight as well as the scientific expertise necessary to fix some of the problems that appear to be inherent in CNS drug development and provide better options for pharma companies and patients alike.

3.4.2 *ADNI: The Prototype Precompetitive Collaboration*

Learning from precompetitive collaborations is a translational approach to promoting innovation, furthering scientific advancements, and increasing productivity throughout the pharmaceutical spectra. Drug companies are forced to manage patent expirations, diminishing market shares, and the recognition that research for drug development has failed to advance a sufficient amount of new drugs through the pipeline. Precompetitive collaborations provide the ability to share research costs among organizations with similar goals to advance research in a specific field. While there have been numerous examples of precompetitive collaborations recently, perhaps it is best illustrated in the 2004 creation of the Alzheimer's Disease Neuroimaging Initiative (ADNI), a public–private partnership involving 20 or so companies working together with academic and government partners. The ADNI is engaged in an effort to bridge gaps in drug discovery and clinical trial development for Alzheimer's disease (AD) by identifying and standardizing methodologies involving biomarkers. Biomarker profiles following cognitive deficits may allow for the characterization and diagnosis of a pre-dementia form of AD. This could change the current practice of diagnosing, managing, and treating AD, and allow for preventative clinical trials. AD drug development must overcome major hurdles, including the currently incomplete understanding of brain pathology, disease progression and variances; validated tools for the early detection of AD are lacking, which contributes to the absence of preventative treatment options; and the current practice of large clinical trials early in development, which, taken together, contribute to high costs without a guarantee of success or a guidance for decision-making. This great need for therapeutic options coupled with the lack in mechanistic understanding led to the creation of ADNI, a longitudinal natural history study funded through a $67m public–private partnership. Research involving imaging and biofluid biomarkers is conducted at over 57 sites across the US and Canada. Since its inception, it has led to over

100 publications and significantly more abstracts that attempt to improve clinical trials by establishing a world-wide network for clinical AD studies and treatment trials, optimizing, standardizing, and validating biomarker methods. Certain patient level databases have been made publicly available, further contributing to the accumulation and integration of the knowledge gained in this partnership. This translational approach joins the public and private sectors in a way that is able to shorten the timetable for scientific advancement to progress drug development in this area [12].

3.4.3 *Advancing Learning Strategies: Transition from Knowing to Learning Organization*

As pharmaceutical companies, such as BMS, look to bring new medications to the market for harder-to-treat diseases that are both poorly understood and have high variance, there is a low probability that a treatment with a single mechanism of action will be efficacious. Response rates can be as low as 45% with certain medication classes such as anti-virals, thereby mandating the public health necessity of seeking novel mechanisms, while currently employing a variety of therapeutic options. New translational strategies include modeling viral kinetics, collaborations between national laboratories, and leveraging prior data from lead compounds to bridge monotherapy data in order to project exposure–response data in combination therapy [13]. In order to support drug development and approval while optimizing risk-benefit to patients and value in the health care field, drug companies have turned to modeling working groups (MWGs). MWGs are integrated, cross-functional expert teams that define and implement the model based drug development (MBDD) strategies at each decision point, enhancing productivity while fostering innovation.

Integrating this learning from prior studies and modeling into routine practice in discovery and development is a key objective of MBDD. In seeking to optimize clinical trial designs, industry has turned to the translational approach of MBDD, by applying the "learn-confirm" paradigm throughout the research and development process. True MBDD starts in discovery and progresses the compound into preclinical development through the use of modeling PK-PD, biomarkers, and *in vitro* data to facilitate suitable animal studies and then to translate this information in the design of effective clinical trials. One company, Covance, utilized its knowledge of intact pathway across species to test a new therapy target for hypertension and diabetes. Animal models suggested that plasma succinic acid (SA) levels may be a biomarker for these conditions, and that GPR91 was a candidate target. However, upon conducting studies, GPR91 antagonism produced no significant differences in serum SA detected in normal, hypertensive, and diabetic humans. GPR91 program was placed on hold pending additional data allowing a clear go/no go decision and reprioritization of resources to other portfolio candidates [14].

3.4.4 *Bioinformatics for Biosamples*

There is a growing appreciation that one of the most valuable data sources for biomedical discoveries is derived from human samples already accumulated in academic, government, and company laboratories throughout the world. This is indicated in the growing number of industry–academic translational medicine partnerships as well as government-supported initiatives such as the Clinical and Translational Science Awards (CTSA) in the United States and the Seventh Framework Programme (FP7) of the EU with its emphasis on translating research for human health.

An example of one company that has instituted a very comprehensive and integrated bioinformatics program to manage biosample data is the pharma conglomerate of Johnson & Johnson. It has established translational and biomarker departments and implemented an effective knowledge management framework including building a data warehouse and associated data mining applications. The implemented resource is built from open source systems such as i2b2 and GenePattern. The system has been deployed across multiple therapeutic areas within the various pharmaceutical companies that comprise J&J, and are being used actively to integrate and mine internal and public data to support drug discovery and development decisions such as indication selection and trial design in a TM setting. Results show that the established system allows scientists to quickly re-validate hypotheses or generate new ones with the use of an intuitive graphical interface. The implemented resource can serve as the basis of precompetitive sharing and mining of studies involving samples from human subjects, thus enhancing understanding of human biology and pathophysiology and ultimately leading to more effective treatment of diseases which represent unmet medical needs [10].

3.4.5 *Imaging-Based Therapeutic Delivery Strategies*

Despite significant diagnostic and therapeutic advances achieved in the last few decades, atherosclerosis is still one of the leading causes of morbidity and mortality worldwide. Until recently, the hemodynamic characteristics of the lesion prevailed over other aspects of the atherosclerosis pathobiologic process. However, it is now well established that independent of the degree of stenosis, other characteristics of the atherosclerosis process, such as endothelial dysfunction, plaque inflammatory activity, platelet agreeability, and neovascularization, are important to determine the progression and complications of the human atherosclerosis plaque.

Against this backdrop, it is paramount that critical events in the atherosclerosis process are imaged at the molecular level, even before a flow-limiting lesion develops. In atherosclerosis and other vascular diseases, molecular imaging provides a personalized insight of the disease-specific biological events, enables novel non-invasive strategies for individualized risk assessment, and facilitates monitoring of highly targeted therapies. Moreover, new imaging technologies targeting specific vascular receptors and development of site-specific delivery methods have expanded the molecular imaging spectrum from a lone diagnostic tool to a mode of therapeutic intervention. In this context, theragnostics, defined as the fusion of diagnosis and therapeutics, is well exemplified by emerging vascular imaging modalities in which highly specific and personalized interventions are delivered using structural, functional, and genomic expressions of the disease. The general goal of an imaging-based therapeutic delivery system is to visualize and control the delivery of a therapeutic agent to a disease-specific region of interest to improve efficacy while reducing unwanted side effects. The principle is to control drug action in the targeted area by an external energy field such as light, neutron beam, magnetic field, or mechanical acoustic energy [15].

SONODRUGS is an integrated project (IP) partly funded by the Nanosciences, Nanotechnologies, Materials and New Production Technologies (NMP) program of the European Commission's 7th Framework that is putting this promising research into practice by developing novel drug delivery technologies for localized treatment of cardiovascular disease and cancer. SONODRUGS develops drug delivery concepts where drug release can be triggered by focused ultrasound induced pressure or temperature stimuli within the diseased tissue. New drug loaded nanocarriers will be designed for tailored drug delivery systems that respond to either of the two stimuli. Medical imaging, i.e., magnetic resonance imaging and ultrasound imaging, will be used to guide, follow, and quantify the drug delivery process. Therapy efficacy using different drug delivery systems will be assessed *in vitro* and subsequently in preclinical studies. Starting from research on a broad range of materials and drugs, two nanocarriers will be finally selected, optimized, and produced on a pilot scale in combination with image-guided delivery tools and methods [16].

Ultrasound, in particular, has significant advantages in becoming the ideal imaging method to deliver a therapeutic intervention. It is the most commonly used non-invasive diagnostic imaging modality. Ultrasound imaging systems are portable and they provide real-time imaging while avoiding hazardous radiation. Moreover, ultrasound is the only non-invasive imaging modality in which multiple human studies have demonstrated the feasibility, efficacy, and prognostic value of using acoustic energy to facilitate fibrinolysis (thrombus sonolysis) and improve drug delivery into tissues and cells [15].

3.5 Future Directions

What does the future hold for TM in the industrial realm? Clearly, the vitality of the TM movement in the public sector bodes well for continued interest on the part of industry with growth spurred by increasing support from government agencies worldwide, particularly in biomarker research. There is a keen appreciation that a translational approach to R&D is a key to efficiently taking advantage of breakthrough technology to achieve both better productivity and better products. In June, 2010 NIH Director Francis Collins and FDA Commissioner Margaret Hamburg co-wrote an article in the New England Journal of Medicine in which they discussed their "shared vision of personalized medicine and the scientific and regulatory structure needed to support its growth.... To make progress, the NIH and the FDA will invest in advancing translational and regulatory science..." [17]. FDA's Critical Path Initiative (CPI) has stated its intention to make broader use of translational science, which is one reason why FDA's Office of Translational Sciences has served in the past as the coordination locus for CPI activities at the agency [7]. The NIH is re-organizing to create NCATS, the National Center for the Acceleration of Translational Sciences, scheduled to be operational in 2012, but remains subject to the vagaries of congressional funding. For its part, the EU's Innovative Medicines Initiative (IMI) has delineated four target areas, one of which is efficacy, and under that banner it highlighted the need to "stimulate translational medicine." This enthusiasm and commitment is shared by industry as the prevalence and expanse of industry collaborations to advance the field of personalized medicines was recently demonstrated by a Tufts CSDD study of approximately 20 major pharma and biotech companies (see Table 3.2) [18].

As always, economics guides the direction of industry investment decisions and resource commitments. The economics of the main TM business segments look attractive at a time when the economic environment in general looks less so. TM and allied fields have the potential to re-energize flagging business prospects. Global biomarkers market is expected to grow to $22bn by 2015, and perhaps as much $34bn by the year 2017 according to the Global Industry Analysts, Inc. (GIA) report [6]. The medical-imaging market in the United States — including ultrasound, magnetic resonance imaging (MRI), radiography and mammography, and computed tomography (CT) — will experience CAGRs of between 9 and 14% for the different market segments, bringing the worth of the market overall to an estimated $11.4bn in 2012, according to a new report by BCC Research, Medical Imaging: Equipment and Related Products. At the same time, a host of developments are taking place in genomics and molecular research that are likely to boost the bioinformatics industry, in conjunction with increasing

R&D investments by various companies and government support. The bioinformatics market will begin posting higher growth rate in most countries. RNCOS's new report "Global Bioinformatics Market Outlook," estimates that the market for bioinformatics will surge at a CAGR of nearly 26% during 2011–2013 to reach a value of around US$6.2bn by 2013.

In the face of government collaboration and coordination of the foundational research and necessary regulatory science, as well as the favorable market predictions for TM business segments, the likelihood of an industrial response geared toward more cost-effective, patient-centered R&D of personalized medicines is almost inevitable in the current healthcare environment. This is good news indeed as industry eagerly anticipates the day when the US personalized medicine market alone with an 11% annual growth rate could reach an estimated $450bn by 2015 [4]. In a world of apparently limitless unmet medical needs and very limited funding resources, hopefully the investment in TM will be money well spent. However, for personalized medicine to reach the goal, in the short-term, of becoming a realistic option for advancing the practice of medicine within the confines of available healthcare system resources, it must pass product-by-product through the crucible of proving its medical utility in the clinic, its potential for routine uptake by the medical community, and its value to third party payers. The speed at which this takes place, and whether indeed it succeeds at all, may well depend initially on the degree of integration at multiple levels of the R&D enterprise of a TM approach focusing on extracting medical tools from the raw materials of basic discovery.

References

1. Using Translational Science to Improve Drug Development, *Tufts CSDD R&D Mgmt. Report* Jan 2011, **6**(1).
2. Nagappa, A.N. (2009). Promise of Translational Medicine: Evidenced-Based Therapeutics, *Pharmabiz.com*, May 12, available at http://www.pharmabiz.com.
3. Feuerstein, G.Z., Chavez, J. (2009). Translational Medicine for Stroke Drug Discovery: The Pharmaceutical Industry Perspective. *Stroke* March **40**(3 Suppl) pp. S121–S125.

4. Milne, C.-P., Kaitin, K.I. (2009). Translational Medicine: An Engine of Change for Bringing New Technology to Community Health. *Science Translational Medicine* 4 November **1**(5: 5). Commentary.
5. Borfitz, D. (2008). Demand Grows for Multi-Purpose Post-Marketing Studies. March 3, available at http://www.barnettclinicalsummit.com/BioIT_Article.aspx?id=72790.
6. Christel, M.D. (2010). Translational Medicine: From Lab to Man. *R&D Directions* April **16**(4) pp. 10–18.
7. Milne, C.-P. (2009). Can Translational Medicine Bring us out of the R&D Wilderness? *Personalized Medicine* September **6**(5) pp. 543–553.
8. Lalonde, R.L. *et al.* (2007). Model-Based Drug Development. *Clinical Pharmacology & Therapeutics* **82** pp. 21–32.
9. Fuchs, V.R., and Sox Jr., H.C. (2001). Physicians' Views of the Relative Importance of Thirty Medical Innovations. Health Aff. (Millwood), **20** pp. 30–42.
10. Szalma, S., Koka, V., Khasanova, T., and Perakslis, E.D. (2010). Effective Knowledge Management in Translational Medicine. *Journal of Translational Medicine* **8** pp. 68.
11. Business Opportunity: Bioinformatics 2009 Update, Invest in Spain, available at http://www.swissbiotech.org.
12. ADNI Website, available at http://adni.loni.ucla.edu/.
13. Gao, M. *et al.* (2010). Chemical Genetics Strategy Identifies an HCV NS5A Inhibitor with a Potent Clinical Effect. *Nature*, **465** pp. 96–100.
14. Turi, T. (2010). Translational Science Strategies to Improve Drug Development. *Covance* Nov. 4 (slide presentation).
15. Eraso, L.H, Reilly, M.P., Sehgal, C., and Mohler, E.R. (2011). Emerging Diagnostic and Therapeutic Molecular Imaging Applications in Vascular Disease. Originally Published Online 10 February *Vascular Medicine* available at http://vmj.sagepub.com/content/16/2/145 (The Online Version of This Article can be Found at: DOI: 10.1177/1358863X10392474 2011 16: 145).
16. SONODRUGS Website, available at http://www.sonodrugs.eu/.
17. Hamburg, M.A., Collins, F.S. (2010). The Path to Personalized Medicine. *New England Journal of Medicine* 22 July, **363**(4) pp. 301–304.
18. Milne, C.-P., Zuckerman, R. (2011). Pharmaceutical Industry Perspectives on the Business Prospects for Personalized Medicine. *Personalized Medicine*, September, **8**(5) pp. 541–550.

Chapter 4

Drivers and Barriers of TM: A Regulatory Perspective

Partha Roy
PAREXEL International, USA
partha.roy@parexel.com

4.1 Introduction

Translational medicine (TM) provides the key bridge (Fig. 4.1) between advances in basic bioscience to clinical medicine that embraces better therapy and improved patient care. It encompasses two primary spaces. First, translation of basic science into drug development tools that can be utilized effectively within the domain of clinical medicine. Second, translating basic science into better understanding of disease etiology and progression, with the objective of discovering, developing, and tailoring new and safer therapeutic options and high-quality care for the individual patient.

Translational Medicine: The Future of Therapy
Edited by James Mittra and Christopher-Paul Milne

ISBN 978-981-4316-99-6 (Hardback), 978-981-4364-84-3 (eBook)
www.panstanford.com

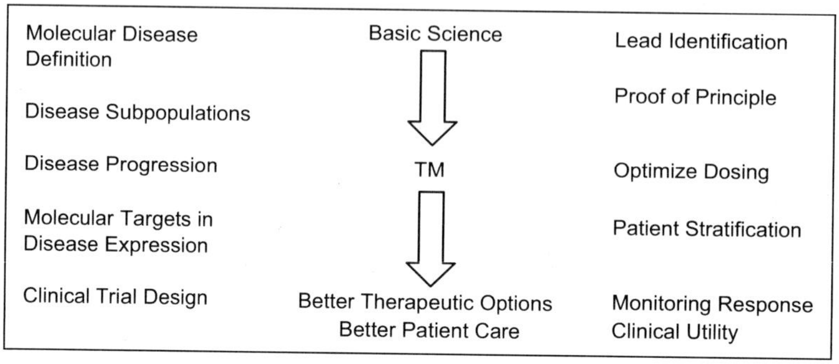

Figure 4.1 Bridging basic science to improved therapeutic options and patient care.

4.2 Drivers of TM

4.2.1 *Drug Development Enterprise*

In the face of skyrocketing healthcare costs and lower rate of success in drug development, there is an urgency to utilize TM for efficient drug development and improved clinical deliverables for the individual patient. However, before we can usefully apply TM to the various stages of drug development, it is imperative that we understand what ails the drug development enterprise. Typically, for development and approval of new drugs, registration trials are conducted in a patient population with a pre-specified range of baseline characteristics. After completion of the registration trials, the data are submitted to the regulatory agencies such as US Food and Drug Administration (FDA) for review of the treatment's benefit–risk ratio. If the benefit–risk ratio is favorable, the treatment will be approved for the studied patient population. Although the process appears simple, there are a lot of underlying uncertainties and the failure rate for new drugs continues to remain high [1,2].

Some relevant examples include:

- Success of only 14% of 39 depression trials in terms of effectiveness [3].
- Rolofylline, a selective A1 receptor antagonist, whose development was dropped after the Phase 3 study data showed

lack of differentiation from placebo in the treatment of acute heart failure [4].

- Lily's decision to not file a New Drug Application for a selective estrogen receptor modulator after completing the pivotal Phase 3 trials, because the clinical profile did not represent a meaningful advancement in the treatment of osteoporosis [4].
- The FDA's non-approval of ximelagatran and subsequent withdrawal of the drug by AstraZeneca from the European market due to severe liver toxicity following longer-term use of the drug [5].
- Post marketing withdrawal of orally administered bromfenac indicated for short-term relief of pain and troglitazone, a treatment for type II diabetes mellitus, due to drug-induced liver toxicity [6].

4.2.2 *Molecular and Genomic Medicine*

Recent biomedical research breakthroughs, including the sequencing of the human genome and a deeper understanding of the molecular underpinnings of disease, have the potential to transform the treatment of disease and the practice of medicine. The integration of genetic information into mainstream medicine to offer personalized treatment choices is increasing, as evidenced by the greater use of pharmacogenetic testing in specialty practices, co-development of drug–device combination pharmacotherapies, recent updates of already approved drug labels and emergence of consumer genomics companies. Personalized medicine has the potential to optimize targeted delivery and dosing of treatments so patients can receive the most benefit with the least amount of risk, cutting out the difficulties of the current trial-and-error process. Identifying patient populations that would most benefit from a therapy is a growing interest in both industry and the regulatory community. Although drug developers want to maximize returns on investment by seeking product labels from the FDA that would provide directions of use of a treatment in the broadest patient population, subgroups in clinical trials, on certain occasions, do show a different benefit/risk profile. This suggests that it is important to identify the patient population in which translation of better benefit/risk profile is most possible.

There are a number of examples of recent FDA approvals that illustrate developments in personalized medicine.

First, BiDil® (isosorbide dinitrate and hydralazine hydrochloride), which is indicated for the treatment of heart failure as an adjunct to standard therapy in self-identified black patients to improve survival, prolong time to hospitalization for heart failure, and improve patient-reported functional status. This was based on a prospectively designed study. Initial identification of a better benefit–risk profile in self-identified black patients was based on retrospective analysis in a study that included self-identified black and white patients (see Fig. 4.2 below). Mechanistically, evidence suggests that black patients with heart failure produce diminished levels of nitric oxide in their coronary and peripheral vasculature,

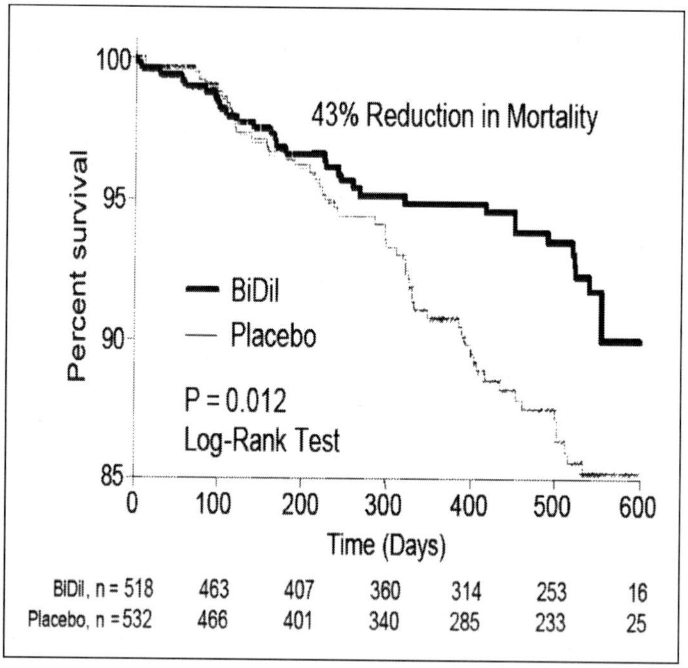

Figure 4.2 Kaplan–Meier plot of time to death by all cause in black patients. Adapted from BiDil package insert, approved on June 23, 2005.

putting them at greater risk than whites [7]. The potential of this combination treatment to increase nitric oxide levels promises to reduce this risk differential. With this logic, it will not be surprising if other drugs with similar mechanisms of action will have similar race-based therapeutic differentials. Here, race is just a crude marker for genetic variations and therefore an interim step toward personalized therapy.

Second, ivacaftor (Kalydeco®), classified as a cystic fibrosis transmembrane conductance regulator (CFTR) potentiator, recently approved by the FDA, is indicated for the treatment of cystic fibrosis (CF) in patients age 6 years and older that have a G551D mutation in the CFTR gene. Kalydeco® is the first available treatment that targets the defective CFTR protein, which is the underlying cause of cystic fibrosis. While announcing the approval of this drug, FDA Commissioner Dr. Margaret A. Hamburg said, "Kalydeco is an excellent example of the promise of personalized medicine — targeted drugs that treat patients with a specific genetic makeup." The FDA reviewed and approved Kalydeco in record time of 3 months, about half the time it takes to approve applications with priority review status that signal an urgency to bring novel highly effective and targeted medications to the patients who would be best positioned to gain benefit. This was approved based on two positive Phase 3 trials in the target population, while a third trial in patients homozygous for the F508del Mutation in the CFTR Gene, the most abundant gating mutation in CF patients, showed lack of efficacy while demonstrating safety consistent with the other trials. This negative trial answers pertinent questions related to its use in the broader patient population, which may occur due to off-label prescribing justified on the basis of the seriousness of the disease. Even if ivacaftor is directed at a responsive G551D subgroup, the drug label provides adequate directions for clinical use with specific language of "not effective in patients with CF who are homozygous for the F508del mutation in the CFTR gene" [8]. This third trial not only provided reasonable amount of safety data in the broader patient population but also provided conclusive evidence that the treatment does not work in the majority of the CF patients. This ultimately will aid physician prescribing practice.

A third example is crizotinib (Xalkori®). On August 26, 2011, the FDA granted conditional and accelerated approval to Xalkori® for the treatment of patients with locally advanced or metastatic non-small cell lung cancer (NSCLC) that is anaplastic lymphoma kinase (ALK)-positive as detected by an FDA-approved test. The FDA approved the Vysis ALK Break-Apart FISH Probe Kit concurrently with the crizotinib approval. This companion diagnostic test is designed to detect rearrangements of the ALK gene in NSCLC. The crizotinib approval was based on response rates of 50% and 61% from 255 ALK-rearranged NSCLC patients enrolled in two single-arm trials. It took only 4 years from the discovery of *ALK* rearrangement in NSCLC to the approval of crizotinib, the first ever ALK inhibitor, for the treatment of *ALK*-rearranged NSCLC. Within the last decade, the important discovery of activating mutations in the kinase domain of the epidermal growth factor receptor (*EGFR*) gene heralded the era of molecular targeted therapy in NSCLC. Crizotinib development was critically based on a fluorescence *in situ* hybridization assay, developed by two of the crizotinib Phase 1 sites [9]. This is a good success story of TM working to accelerate development of a highly effective targeted medicine for the patient population most likely to benefit.

4.2.2.1 Pharmacogenomic information in drug labels

Over the past decade, the FDA has been a strong advocate for the incorporation of pharmacogenomics information in the product label, in order to make drugs more safe and effective for the individual patient or a specific patient population. Regulatory authorities in the three major geographic regions are increasingly adding PGx information to label updates of approved drugs, as well as incorporating PGx into their regulatory review of new products. There are three important considerations that influence the incorporation of PGx information in product labels: (1) generation of guidelines on evidentiary considerations for PGx to be included in the product labels; (2) the section(s) of the product label where PGx information is included, and; (3) clinical utility of the new information and how professional medical organizations, individual physicians and third-party payers weigh the evidence to instigate a change in medical practice. The goal is to ensure a degree of consensus amongst all stakeholders (patients, healthcare providers, drug developers, and regulators) about how to accurately interpret and implement the information to positively influence medical decision-making. A few prominent examples, spanning various indications, include *6-mercaptopurine* (6-MP) linking TPMT and 6-MP induced myelosuppression; *irinotecan* (Camptosar®) associated with UGT1A1 mutations with increased susceptibility to neutropenia; *warfarin* (Coumadin®) linking variable dose requirements with CYP2C9–VKORC1 combination genotypes; *carbamazepine* (Tegretol®) associating variants in the gene HLA-B*1502 with increased risk of developing life-threatening skin reactions; *abacavir* (Ziagen®) linking HLA-B*5701 with higher risk of a hypersensitivity reaction; and *clopidogrel* (Plavix®) impacted by CYP2C19 poor metabolizer status with a diminished antiplatelet response and higher cardiovascular event rates than CYP2C19 extensive metabolizers (see FDA Table of Pharmacogenomic Biomarkers in Drug Labels, http://www.fda.gov/Drugs/ScienceResearch/ResearchAreas/Pharmacogenetics/ucm083378.htm).

Besides incorporating pharmacogenomics information in drug labels, over the last few years the FDA has taken a leadership role on the scientific front and build the infrastructure necessary to support the development of personalized targeted therapies, most immediately through investments in regulatory science, clarification of FDA policies, a reorganization of leadership, and engagement of physicians, patients, and their advocacy groups. One such example of the FDA promoting innovation through regulatory science is in the area of stem cells. Scientists at the FDA's Center for Biologics Evaluation and Research (CBER), in collaboration with NIH, the National Institute of Standards and Technology (NIST), and academia, are developing new methods to evaluate stem cells using a variety of advanced analytic methods that compare the cells' characteristics when grown in a dish to how they change when placed in an animal. The knowledge gained from these studies, including the cells' characteristics and how they change, can contribute to the development of safe and effective embryonic stem (ES) cell-based products for humans and will be used to create advanced tools and processes for evaluating how ES cell-based products planned for humans will perform.

Another example where the FDA is trying to make a difference is with the development of companion diagnostics, i.e. the tests that are used to determine whether a particular therapy may work for a particular patient. A good example is the recent approval of Crizotinib, approved for locally advanced or metastatic non-small cell lung cancer (NSCLC) that is anaplastic lymphoma kinase-positive as detected by an FDA-approved test. The FDA issued the draft guidance entitled *In Vitro Companion Diagnostic Devices* on July 14, 2011, to communicate to industry how the FDA defines these devices and to assist sponsors in understanding the Agency's perspective on them. As a follow on to the *In Vitro Companion Diagnostic Devices* guidance, the FDA is also developing a draft guidance outlining strategies for clinical trial design and regulatory considerations for co-developing a novel companion diagnostic and therapy simultaneously, where the approval and subsequent use of the therapy would incorporate a requirement for the diagnostic test. This draft guidance will include recommendations for the strategic use of biomarkers for patient selection and screening, as well as clinical trial designs that allow for ethical patient selection strategies. The FDA is also producing an internal plan for how it will review applications using co-development strategies for product development to accompany both guidances and ensure the Agency meets the special needs of these types of products in a timely way.

4.2.3 *Emphasis on Preclinical Pharmacology*

For a long time there has been a missing link between preclinical information and the understanding of human pharmacology and individual variations in clinical response to therapeutic interventions. There is a need for a new discipline that can promote pharmacology-based drug development and effectively link preclinical pharmacology to human pharmacology in a quantitative manner. The current lack of systematic translation of nonclinical findings is exemplified by a relatively recent example. The first-in-man Phase 1 clinical trial with the monoclonal antibody TGN1412, which ended in the near-death inflammatory response called "cytokine storm," prompted scientists and regulators to look back and investigate whether this disaster could have been avoided from the information generated in pre-clinical testing. The animal safety testing revealed that the preclinical safety testing was conducted in a non-responsive species with improper antigen presentation. In particular, little attention was paid to understanding the CD28 binding differences, and subsequent signal transduction, between human and cynomolgus monkey. There was more focus on the knowledge that TGN1412 binds with high affinity to a 6 amino acid epitope on an extracellular loop of the CD28 molecule that is entirely conserved between man and macaques. Subsequently, the drug developer may have incorrectly considered cynomolgus macaques to be the most relevant species for pre-clinical safety testing.

Most drugs fail due to lack of clinical efficacy. This is difficult to comprehend considering major advances in basic science supporting target identification, lead generation, and preclinical pharmacology models. Predictions for novel interventions in preclinical stages of development often suffer from lack of understanding of validation in preclinical research and an overly optimistic reliance on a narrow piece of favorable evidence that sways decision-makers to promote drug candidates for clinical testing. For example, in the case of AstraZeneca's failed stroke drug NXY-059, use of normotensive rodents in preclinical development may have led to spurious predictions of clinical activity [10]. One widely recognized target for the development of drugs to treat Alzheimer's disease is the prevention of amyloid-beta accumulation in the brains of Alzheimer patients. Semagacestat, a gamma secretase inhibitor Eli Lily was developing, was screened and designed to target amyloid-β production and expected to be effective against dementia. However, results from two long-term Phase 3 studies showed it did not slow disease progression and was associated with worsening of clinical measures of cognition and the ability to perform activities of daily living. Retrospectively, it is noted that trials were launched on the basis of molecular, rather than behavioral, endpoints; which raises questions about the validity of preclinical investigations in making clinical generalizations [11].

4.3 Impact of TM on Regulatory Decision Making and Barriers to TM

The FDA is increasingly utilizing concepts of TM into regulatory decision making to supplement the information generated from confirmatory trials. Advances in this area are providing unique opportunities for the FDA to adopt a risk-based regulatory approach toward drug approval that is increasingly driven by concepts from TM. Over the last few years, the FDA has been increasingly relying on biomarkers/surrogates and pharmacometric approaches to review and approve new drug applications. This has been to facilitate the streamlining of drug development based on translational strategies and mechanistic understanding, with the expectation that it will lead to significant cost savings and reduction of development time and, at the same time, get novel and much-needed therapies quickly to patients. Qualified biomarkers can enrich clinical trials by demonstrating benefits, establishing unmet medical needs, and identifying patients with a predisposition to adverse events.

For example, the utility of hemodynamics in assessing treatment response in children with pulmonary arterial hypertension (PAH) that are unable to perform exercise testing, has recently attracted considerable attention as an alternative to the gold standard of exercise capacity to determine a medicine's efficacy (see FDA Advisory Committee Briefing Document for *Revatio* 2010). Work recently carried out by both Pfizer and the FDA indicates that drug-induced changes in exercise capacity were associated with drug-induced changes in pulmonary vascular resistance index (PVRI) in patients with PAH. This suggests that drug-induced changes in PVRI might be used to make an informed assessment of treatment benefit of *Revatio* (*sildenafil*) for PAH in children of all ages. The relationship seems to be consistent across drugs of several classes and in control groups. This highlights the effective utilization of a practical clinical surrogate.

Evidence supporting clinical utility becomes a key driver for clinical adoption and personalized medicine. However, the question boils down to how much evidence one needs and how that evidence should be generated. It is important to keep in mind that the majority of evidence generated to support the clinical utility of a drug and companion diagnostic has occurred incrementally over time [12]. Incremental benefits should not be held against widespread adoption. Clinical utility is often a matter of judgment; depending on a stakeholder's perspective of the supporting evidence. That certainly does not mean that we should not strive for a higher level of evidence to establish clinical validity and support clinical implementation for a positive public health outcome. Evidence generation leads to the much-needed discussion of study design (e.g., enrichment design) and regulatory framework (pre- vs. post-approval) that create opportunities for the generation of useful data [13]. This can potentially facilitate improved integration of drug and diagnostic tests into clinical practice.

The recent example of slow uptake of genetic testing for warfarin in the clinic illustrates this struggle. The label for warfarin has been updated with biomarker information, which needed the clinical practice to change in order to be comprehensively adopted (http://www.accessdata.fda.gov/drugsatfda_docs/label/2011/009218s107lbl.pdf). However, very few patients get tested for VKORC1 and CYP2C9 when prescribed warfarin, despite much observational evidence of clinical utility of this information for optimum dosing. In a recent observational pharmacogenomic-warfarin dosing study led by Medco and Mayo Clinic, researchers found that hospitalizations due to any cause, as well as due to blood clots or excessive bleeding, for heart patients taking warfarin dropped by approximately 30% when genetic information was available to doctors [14]. However, critics raised the possibility that the 30% reduction in hospitalizations in the study may have been due to the effect of closer attention to the patient rather than the effect of genotyping prior to dosing [15]. Experts in the field wondered whether we could achieve similar goals simply by using a dosing algorithm that takes age, gender, body surface area, and early INR response into account. These are valid arguments considering the cost of genetic testing and the feasibility of obtaining the test results in real-time without significant inconvenience to patients and health-care providers. In addition, there are enough conflicting reports from clinical trials, including prospective randomized controlled investigations, to polarize this debate. The first randomized prospective controlled trial to compare genotype-guided dosing to standard empirical dosing has produced negative results of no difference in proportion of out-of-range INRs between intervention and control groups. However, the same study enumerated several key findings to support the use of genetic testing that have been discussed in detail by Lesko [16].

Clinical data seems to follow a hierarchy of evidence, with meta-analyses and randomized controlled trials constituting the highest level of evidence and expert opinion being the lowest [17]. This has been the case with *abacavir* hypersensitivity, where clinical adoption has been relatively rapid and widespread for HLA-B*5701 prescreening to identify patients for the at-risk allele prior to initiating therapy. Positive and unambiguous data from a randomized controlled trial [18] provided evidence of clinical utility, which not only led to speedy adoption into clinical guidelines but also paved the way for positive reimbursement decisions from insurance companies and rapid acceptance by both the physician and patient communities [19]. We also often see that having a strong causal relationship between genetic evidence and clinical outcome is not enough to encourage clinical adoption.

4.4 Concluding Remarks

Experience at the FDA suggests that failure to utilize prior knowledge about the drug and the disease often accounts for trial failure, which is either lack of differentiation with placebo or identification of unanticipated adverse effects. TM can make the drug development process more quantitative and science-driven; provide important clues and opportunities to look at the early data and make any necessary corrections in the confirmatory stage, such as how to get the correct dose for the most appropriate patient. The National Center for Toxicological Research (NCTR) is playing an important role in conducting FDA mission-critical, peer-reviewed, translational research to develop a scientifically sound basis for regulatory decisions and reduce risks associated with FDA-regulated products. This NCTR research evaluates the biological effects of potentially toxic chemicals or microorganisms; defines the complex mechanisms that govern their toxicity; aids in understanding critical biological events in the expression of toxicity; and develops new scientific tools and methods to improve assessment of human exposure, susceptibility, and risk [20].

In the United States, drug-induced liver injury (DILI) is now the leading cause of acute liver failure (ALF), exceeding all other causes combined. Because of this, DILI has been identified by the FDA's Critical Path Initiatives [21] as a key area of focus in a concerted effort to broaden the agency's knowledge for better evaluation tools and safety biomarkers.

In August 2007, the FDA entered a 2-year Cooperative Research and Development Agreement (CRADA) with Entelos, a leader in predictive biosimulation, to develop a "virtual patient" computer model simulation to predict whether new drugs will produce DILI. The goal is to use this *in silico* platform to guide the development of clinical biomarkers and preclinical assays to identify patient types and drug combinations that increase the risk of liver injury. In addition to the CRADA, the FDA issued a contract with Entelos, Inc, in September 2008 to perform an exhaustive review of the scientific literature and produce the first implementation step of the computer model, describing the currently known and hypothesized mechanisms for DILI (ref: FDA website; http://www.fda.gov/aboutfda/partnershipscollaborations/publicprivatepartnershipprogram/ucm231122.htm).

There are several venues for TM to revolutionize drug development enterprises by applying advanced tools to optimize dosing, identifying the right patient population for drugs in development, and providing the means to apply informed clinical trial design to answer the most pertinent questions. Together, these can help to reduce attrition, minimize failure and appropriately define clinical utility.

References

1. Eichler, H.G., *et al.* (2010). New drug approval success rate in Europe in 2009, *Nat. Rev. Drug Discov.* **9**, 355–356.

2. DiMasi, J.A., *et al.* (2010). Trends in risks associated with new drug development: success rates for investigational drugs. Clinical Pharmacology & Therapeutics **87** (3), 272–277.
3. Hooper, M. and Amsterdam, J.D. (1998). *Do clinical trials reflect drug potential? A review of FDA evaluation of new antidepressants.* Paper Presented at Annu. NCDEU Meeting., 39th, Boca Raton, Fla., 11–14 June.
4. Honig, P. and Lalonde, R. (2010). The economics of drug development: a grim reality and a role for clinical pharmacology, *Clin. Pharmacol. Therap.* **87**(3), pp. 247–251.
5. Lee, WM, *et al.* (2005) Hepatic findings in long-term clinical trials of ximelagatran, *Drug Saf.* **28**(4), pp. 351–70.
6. Goldkind, L. and Laine, L. (2006). A systematic review of NSAIDs withdrawn from the market due to hepatotoxicity: lessons learned from the bromfenac experience, *Pharmacoepidemiol. Drug Saf.* 2006 **15**(4), pp. 213–220.
7. Stein, C.M., *et al.* (1997). Vasodilation in black Americans: attenuated nitric oxide-mediated responses, *Clin. Pharmacol. Therap.,* **62**(4), pp. 436–443.
8. Kalydeco label at Drugs@FDA: http://www.accessdata.fda.gov/scripts/cder/drugsatfda/index.cfm?fuseaction=Search.DrugDetails.
9. Sai-Hong Ignatius, Ou. (2011). Crizotinib: a novel and first-in-class multitargeted tyrosine kinase inhibitor for the treatment of anaplastic lymphoma kinase rearranged non-small cell lung cancer and beyond, *Drug Des Devel Ther.* 5, pp. 471–485.
10. Bath, P.M.W., *et al.* (2009). Effects of NXY-059 in experimental stroke: an individual animal meta-analysis, *Br. J. Pharmacol.,* **157**, pp. 1157–1171.
11. Kimmelman, J. and London, A.J. (2011). Predicting harms and benefits in translational trials: ethics, evidence and uncertainty, *PLoS Med* **8** (3), p. e1001010.
12. Woodcock, J. (2010). Assessing the clinical utility of diagnostics used in drug therapy, *Clin. Pharmacol. Therap.* **88**, pp. 765–773.
13. Temple, R. (2010). Enrichment of Clinical Study Populations, *Clin. Pharmacol. Therap.* **88**(6), pp. 774–778.
14. Epstein, R.S., *et al.* (2010). Warfarin genotyping reduces hospitalization rates: results from the MM-WES (Medco-Mayo Warfarin Effectiveness Study), *J Am Coll Cardiol,* **55**, pp. 2804–2812.
15. Turna, R. (2010). Clinical utility of PGx-guided Warfarin dosing not proven in Mayo-Medco study, reviewer concludes at cardiology meeting, *Yahoo Finance News.*

16. Lesko, L.J. (2008). The critical path of Warfarin dosing: finding an optimal dosing strategy using pharmacogenetics, *Clin. Pharmacol. Therap.* **84**(3), pp. 303–305.
17. Harbour, R. and Miller, J.A. (2001). A new system for grading recommendations in evidence based guidelines, *BMJ* **323**, pp. 334–336.
18. Mallal, S., *et al.* (2008). PREDICT-1 Study Team. HLA-B*5701 screening for hypersensitivity to abacavir, *NEJM* **358**, pp. 568–579.
19. Lesco, L.J. and Zineh, I. (2010). DNA, drugs and chariots: on a decade of pharmacogenomics at the US FDA, *Pharmacogenomics*, **11**(4), pp. 507–512.
20. NCTR Strategic Plan, available at https://www.hsdl.org/?view&did=28370).
21. FDA (2006) *Critical path opportunities report*, US Department of Health and Human Services, March, 2006, http://www.fda.gov/downloads/ScienceResearch/SpecialTopics/CriticalPathInitiative/CriticalPathOpportunitiesReports/UCM077254.pdf.

Chapter 5

Developing an Evaluation Model for Translational Medicine Research Programs

Jim Jackson
University of Edinburgh, UK

5.1 Introduction and Background

Translational medicine and translational medicine research (TMR) has been gaining increasing recognition over the past decade. It is referred to directly in a number of funding programmes [1,2], and in Scotland there has been a major public–private collaboration called the Translational Medicine Research Initiative (http://www.tmri.co.uk/). There are now courses and training programs in TMR, and an Institute for Translational Medicine and Therapeutics at the University of Pennsylvania (http://www.itmat.upenn.edu/).

Although there is much currency in the concept of TMR, there have also been voices of caution. The modest success in introducing new therapies as a result of TMR has been attributed to fragmentation and the lack of a global response to the challenges of putting

Translational Medicine: The Future of Therapy
Edited by James Mittra and Christopher-Paul Milne

ISBN 978-981-4316-99-6 (Hardback), 978-981-4364-84-3 (eBook)
www.panstanford.com

TMR into practice [3]. TMR has been described as "fashionable," and one author has stated "most activities under the umbrella "translational medicine" are pretentious and reflect phraseology, thus just wishful thinking" [4]. Others have pointed to translational research overlapping systems biology, experimental medicine, and experimental therapeutics with clinical pharmacology playing a central role [5].

It is timely to both address the question of what TMR actually is and construct a working definition that could be used in the development of an evaluation model for TMR projects. It is important to recognize that the broad scope and long timescales over which the benefits of TMR might expect to be observed poses a difficulty for any evaluative model. In order to try and manage this complexity, I borrow concepts from systems theory in building the evaluation model. A small scale translational research program, in which the final reports were available, was used to pilot the evaluation model.

There are a number of reasons why is it important to evaluate TMR. First, with increasing competition for public funding, biomedical research has to demonstrate its cost-effectiveness to public funding bodies [6,7]. Pharmaceutical companies must also make strategic R&D decisions regarding funding and portfolio management at a time when there is a shortage of new, innovative products coming through their pipelines [8], and small companies face problems accessing venture capital [9,10].

Furthermore, the escalating costs of drug development is a continuing challenge for the pharmaceutical sector [11,12], and TMR has been proposed as a key response to both this and the pipeline problem. Other responses include mergers and acquisitions and strategic alliances/partnerships [13–16].

Although TMR has been proposed as a new approach to accelerating drug discovery, it has not yet been subjected to full evaluative scrutiny. It is not clear how it should be evaluated, however, because of the broad range of definitions and approaches to TMR; the multiple and complex stages between basic research and the introduction of a new medical treatment; and the continual changes that are taking place within the pharmaceutical sector. It is also important for any proposed evaluative model to consider the impact of TMR on the disease burden and public health both nationally and internationally [17–19].

A further point to note is that one of the potential obstacles to the introduction of a new therapy is the need for regulatory approval for safety, efficacy, and in some countries cost-effectiveness [20]. This can add significantly to the costs of the pharmaceutical industry and slow down the introduction of new therapies [21–23]. One of TMR's key objectives is to identify and validate reliable biomarkers for efficacy and toxicity that will enable early decisions to be made about whether to progress a therapy to clinical trial [11].

In developing an evaluation model for TMR, four important research questions are considered:

1. Is there any consensus on the defining features of TMR?
2. If there is little agreement on the definition of TMR, what consequences does this have for its evaluation?
3. Is it possible to develop a viable evaluation model for TMR that could be applied consistently?
4. What implications might the development and piloting of a TMR evaluation model for a single case have for the future evaluation of TMR projects?

This chapter provides an in-depth description and analysis of the pilot evaluation model. By highlighting the key differences in how TMR has been described, and constructing a workable definition, this chapter contributes to greater precision and understanding of what the key features of TMR are and hopefully provide some clarity that the field urgently requires [24–26]. By piloting an evaluation model, and demonstrating how new TMR initiatives might be evaluated, this chapter provides a starting point for thinking about the development of more substantial evaluative models in the future.

5.2 Preparing to Build the Evaluation Model

An extensive literature search, conducted by the author in early 2010, did not identify any established evaluation models for TMR against which it would be possible to assess current research projects. It was therefore necessary to build a new evaluation model. Since the goal was to specifically evaluate the translational features of TMR, the model excludes various questions that would be expected within standard research program evaluation; such as questions about the appropriateness of the methods, procedures for minimizing bias, and whether the interpretation of data was reasonable.

The following methodological steps were undertaken by the author to build and pilot the model.

1. Extensive literature search for definitions of TMR. In order to identify definitions or descriptions of TMR, literature searches were carried out in Medline and PubMed. The top 20 articles from the *Journal of Translational Medicine* were also checked. This resulted in some 200 articles whose abstracts were read whenever possible. From these articles, a list of definitions was prepared. In addition, articles were selected which contained descriptions, explanations, reviews, and assessments of TMR. It was these articles, and those from which the definitions had been taken, which were used to build a new working definition of TMR from which the evaluation model would be developed.
2. Interviews with both practitioners of TMR (2 interviews in total) and funders of TMR projects (5 interviews in total). Most of the interviews were face-to-face, one was by telephone and one was by email. The funders that were interviewed included: the Chief Scientist Office, Scottish Government Health Department; the UK Medical Research Council; the Translational Medicine Research Initiative and the Wellcome Trust.
3. In-depth analysis of the different definitions of TMR and subsequent development of an evaluation model for TMR in Scotland.
4. Piloting the evaluation model against specific projects that were funded in 2007 by the Biomedical and Therapeutic Research Committee of the Chief Scientist Office (CSO), Scottish Government, under the Experimental Medicine – Translational Medicine Research Grants [27].

In 2007, the Scottish Government Health Directorate's CSO funded 14 translational medicine research projects. These studies had been completed and the final reports were in the public domain when this study began. Although these were small projects and do not necessarily represent the scale of larger TMR initiatives, they were chosen as exemplars of TMR that could be compared with a descriptive definition of TMR and used to pilot the evaluation model. The aim of the *Experimental Medicine — Translational Medicine Research Grants* scheme was to encourage translation of basic research findings to have an impact on diagnosis, treatment, or prevention. The 14 funded projects covered a diverse range of topics including cell biomarkers for oocyte and embryo development competence, risk genes for dyslexia, differential proteomics of the normal brain and gliomas, and investigation into the genetic determinants of corticosteroid resistance.

5.3 Identifying and Analysing Definitions of TMR

Defining TMR for the purpose of developing an evaluation model was not straightforward for a number of reasons. First, TMR crosses organizational boundaries (academia, pharmaceutical companies, biotech companies, clinical practice, and regulatory agencies), and each can have a different view as to what TMR is. Second, TMR is multidisciplinary, including genomics, cell and pathway biology, physiology, experimental medicine, clinical studies, etc., so there is a diverse and complex disciplinary nomenclature to contend with. Finally, different stakeholders (analysts, funders, practitioners, users) may emphasize different features of TMR to suit their own particular interest in the field.

Twenty two different definitions were discovered in the literature search and could be broadly categorized in three ways.

First, there were a number of definitions that focused on TMR as being "applied basic science." An early example from 2002 stated, "translational research can be simply defined as a process of determining a treatment solely on the basis of molecular biological characteristics" [28]. A more recent example defines TMR as "the translation of genomic and functional biology discoveries into clinical practice" [29]. These short definitions lead to an obvious question — which molecular, biological, or genomic characteristics? A partial answer is found in some of the longer definitions. For example, Fontanarosa and DeAngelis define TMR as "studies of novel discoveries that advance the understanding of disease mechanisms and provide insights that may prove useful in improving the diagnosis, treatment, and prevention of common diseases and conditions" [30]. This example illustrates how TMR looks backwards to improve understanding of underlying disease pathology, and forwards to the improvement of diagnosis, treatment, or prevention. The longer definitions also tend to be more specific about objectives intermediate to basic research and new therapies, such as "biomarkers, clinical methods, clinical technologies, and study designs" [31], and "patient selection, dosing regime, and disease segment" [25].

Second, a number of the definitions implied that TMR is a journey from basic science through to clinical application [32,33]. However, others have emphasized that TMR should be a two-way process [34–36], where clinical observations generate hypotheses to be tested at the biological level. It has been suggested that the tendency for descriptions of TMR to be more from "bench to bedside" than "bedside to bench" may be due to a hierarchy of credibility where basic science is seen to have greater status than clinical practice [37]. A patient-oriented focus has also been identified as being important in ensuring that innovation reaches those who most need it [38].

Third, a final category encompasses those definitions that view TMR as having two or more stages. The National Institutes of Health (NIH) talks about two areas of translation: applying findings from basic research to trials and human studies, and "enhancing the adoption of best practices in the community" [39]. The working definition developed by Rubio *et al.* [36] goes slightly further in describing a stage that explicitly explores the relationship and relevance of population research to laboratory research and vice versa. Woolf [24] has argued for a clearer and more explicit distinction between the first two stages to be recognized. This generated a number of responses from other authors supporting the need for greater clarity, with suggestions for changes in nomenclature such as preclinical research for the first stage and applied clinical research for the second stage [40], or knowledge translation for the second stage [41]. Others have supported not only recognition of different stages of TMR, but also the need for different academic disciplines and skills, such as epidemiology and the study of human behavior [42].

The multiple definitions of TMR confirm that there is a lack of clarity and consensus in how the terms translational medicine and translational research are used. This has profound implications for the development of a TMR evaluation model that can be applied consistently. Conclusions drawn from an evaluation model based on a particular definition are unlikely to be applicable to TMR projects that fall under a different definition. It is therefore important to construct a sufficiently broad definition that encompasses salient features expressed within the different categorizations. Here, we can usefully employ elements from systems thinking.

5.4 Applying Systems Thinking to the Model

An alternative to selecting a single definition of TMR from the literature is to use concepts from systems theory and program evaluation to create a new, broadly applicable definition that takes into account some of the earlier definitions.

One useful systems approach is what is called "soft systems methodology" [43,44]. It consists of repeatedly assessing the context of a phenomenon or problem, drawing up models of purposeful activity, discussing and analysing the models to create a working model, and then using the working model to respond to the phenomenon or problem.

Model building uses the CATWOE mnemonic (described later) to facilitate the creation of a root definition to describe the system under consideration. The key strength of this approach is that is suited to "messy project situations" that do not easily fit with hard organizational boundaries, and where there is less or no need for feedback loops in order for the system to be stable.

The Basic Program Logic Model has been used, *inter alia*, in the United States as part of the evaluation process for public health programs. It is useful in distinguishing inputs, activities, outputs, and

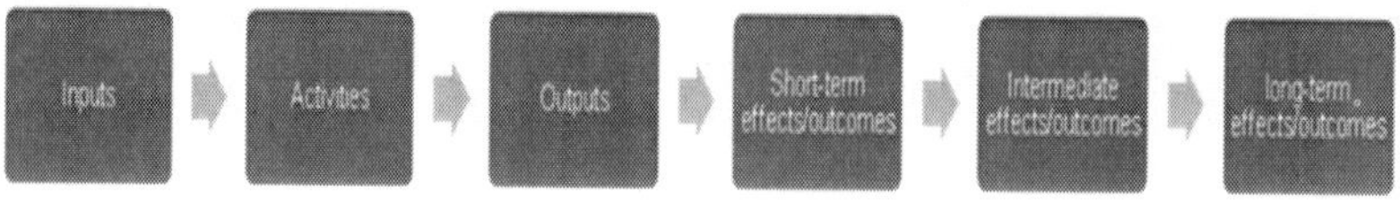

Figure 5.1 Basic Programme Logic Model [46].

outcomes, and it recognizes that outcomes can be further broken down into short-term, intermediate, and long-term. An example of its use can be seen a framework that was developed for the evaluation of HIV/AIDS clinical trials networks [45]. The model is represented in Fig. 5.1.

The first stage in developing a definition of TMR was to review the definitions and selected articles from the literature of TMR and summarize them using the structure of the Basic Program Logic Model. This helped identify the common features of TMR and differences between approaches. This was followed by using soft systems methodology to create a working definition of TMR.

The Basic Program Logic Model analysis of the collected definitions and other selected TMR literature showed that most focus on the outputs — such as "new tools for diagnosis, therapy, and prevention" [47], "novel biomarkers" [48] or "smart early human study design" [4] — from basic, clinical, and discovery research, which are thought necessary to accelerate and improve the process of drug/therapy development. The assumption, common to many definitions, that molecular biology will determine future treatments is well summarized in Saijo's definition [28] — "translational research can be defined simply as the process of determining a treatment solely on the basis of molecular biological characteristics." However, this fails to recognize that TMR is a "bi-directional spectrum" [49] where hypotheses from basic science may originate in clinical observations [50] and epidemiological data [42]. A more sophisticated example of the deterministic molecular biology approach is provided by Webb and Pass [51], who have developed a diagnosis-to-treatment systems model that links the data generated by genomics and proteomics with detecting, typing, staging, treating, and monitoring disease. This model also demonstrates that although it is possible to define TMR simply as

Table 5.1 Use of the CATWOE mnemonic to describe TMR

Mnemonic	Explanation of mnemonic	Mnemonic applied to TMR
C	Customers, beneficiaries, victims, etc.	Patients, health practitioners, and health-care systems
A	Actors	Basic researchers, clinical researchers, funders, pharmaceutical industry, regulators, academia, government
T	Transformation process — include direct object of main activity verb	Developing new therapies from insights created by basic research and feedback from clinical research
W	Weltanschauung — outlook, framework, or image that makes the definition meaningful	"bench to bedside," "bedside to bench" interdependent chain accelerated drug development and innovation
O	Ownership	Dispersed and partially shared
E	Environmental constraints	Funding, skills and abilities of researchers, organization of research effort, capacity for cooperation and multidisciplinary work, requirements of the regulatory agencies

"applying bench-side discoveries in a clinical setting," its description is far more complicated.

The Basic Program Logic Model usefully captures the different emphases from definitions in the broad literature; for example, the development of new research tools [52], the series of processes or complex system that involves, for example, the careers of researchers [53], or the role of regulatory agencies [3,54]. It also recognizes the breadth of TMR that is implied by some authors [48] rather than described [54].

The next step in creating a new working definition of TMR was to use the CATWOE mnemonic as a framework to identify common features that can then be used in root definition as described in soft systems methodology. The use of the CATWOE mnemonic is shown in Table 5.1.

Root definitions try to capture what a system has to do, how it can do it, and why it is done. An initial possible root definition of TMR based on the CATWOE mnemonic and definitions/descriptions taken from the literature (TMR as a *purposeful drug development process)*, might be *Translational medicine research integrates findings from basic and clinical research in order to increase understanding of*

- *pathology of disease,*
- *potential targets for new drugs,*
- *operating systems of new drugs*, and
- *efficacy and safety of new drugs*
- *to accelerate new drug development for patient benefit.*

A working definition, which takes into account data from the interviews with funders (particularly their emphasis on potential benefits to society and the importance of having a broader perspective than simply drug development), and essential features of how translational research needs to be carried out as proposed in the FDA's Critical Path Opportunities Report [55], might be *Translational medicine research is an interdependent chain which integrates findings from basic and clinical research and the different stages of therapy development in order to increase understanding of*

- *mechanisms which maintain health,*
- *pathology of disease,*
- *potential targets of new therapies including drugs, behaviour, and biological products such as stem cells,*
- *operating systems of new therapies, and*
- *efficacy and safety of new therapies*

to accelerate therapy development for the benefit of patients, potential patients, and society.

Translational medicine research is likely to include

- *biomarker development — improving diagnosis, predicting diagnosis, validating the choice of candidate therapies, monitoring the effects of treatment, identifying potential adverse events and safety issues defining patient populations*
- *streamlining clinical trials — phase zero trials, using biomarkers to generate more information especially in phase 1 and 2 trials*

- *bioinformatics — standardisation of trial design and choice of biomarkers, data banks for information sharing, and silica data mining.*

It is possible to continue this iterative process of refining definitions, for example to cover the wider systems perspectives of medical research as a whole, or national/international economies.

The second definition of TMR can be represented diagrammatically with the assistance of the Basic Program Logic Model (Fig. 5.2).

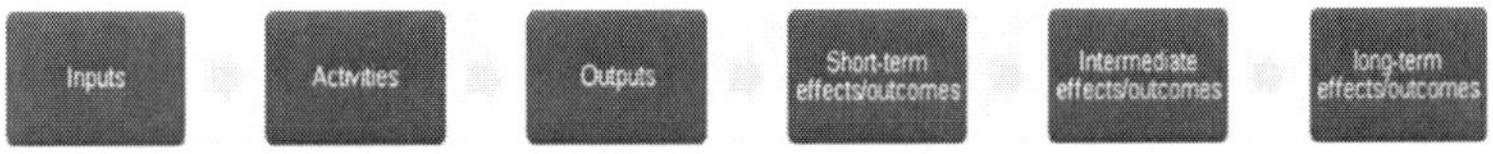

Inputs	Activities	Outputs	Short-term outcomes	Intermediate outcomes	Long-term outcomes
Basic science	Experimentation	Better understanding of pathology and potential treatment targets in humans	Clinical trials of new drugs and devices	Efficacy and toxicity of treatments	Improved patient outcomes
Clinical science	Discovery research	Understanding how new drugs work	New diagnostic tools	More accurate and differential diagnosis	Improved public health
Careers of researchers	Pathway finding	Understanding mechanisms which maintain health	New biomarkers	Regulatory approval	
	Identification of new targets	Potential new drugs	Streamlined clinical trials		
	Use of animal models of disease	Potential biomarkers	Greater use of bioinformatics		
	Early compound or device testing	Scientific innovations			
		New research tools			

Figure 5.2 Stages of translational medicine research incorporated in the "interdependent chain" definition of TMR and the Basic Program Logic Model.

5.5 Building the Evaluation Model

Evaluation is largely about determining value. How might we then determine the value of TMR? First, it is necessary to recognize that the value might be in terms of medical research in general or translational research in particular. For the former, we face the challenge that until recently this has been a relatively under developed area of research because of its sheer complexity. For the latter, it will depend on whether TMR is to be evaluated as an all-encompassing research system, including its infrastructure, judged by its high-level outcomes; a stage or series of stages within the drug or therapy development process; or a tool or methodology that will contribute to improving the effectiveness of translational research.

The following model was designed to generate data that can be used to evaluate TMR as the system described in the Basic Program Logic Model, using the definition of TMR as "an interdependent chain." It could also be selectively used for the evaluation of one or more stages of TMR or its specific tools/methodology. The model has three parts, which are organized around three key questions:

1. To what extent can the research be considered as TMR?
2. Has the research added value to TMR?
3. Does TMR reflect current Scottish health priorities and needs?

The first question asks whether a particular piece of medical research can legitimately be described as translational. The range of definitions has already been described and key differences between them noted. One of the author's interviews with a funder of TMR suggested that there was a great deal of confusion as to the meaning of translational research and that, consequently, many applicants claimed that research was translational without being able to justify that claim. It has also been stated that there is a "paucity of real translational work" [56]. In order to overcome this uncertainty this study uses the "interdependent chain" definition and its diagrammatic representation using the Basic Program Logic Model to create an "is this TMR" checklist. The idea behind the check list was to build a descriptive profile of individual pieces of research in order to see how closely they matched the definition of TMR.

The next step was to consider whether the TMR features of a research study added value to TMR as a whole. This was approached in two ways. The first explored different ways of evaluating medical research, and asked whether there was evaluative criteria that could also be applied to TMR. The second considered the interview subject's response when they were asked to complete the sentence — "translational medicine will be successful if...".

TMR can be thought of as a complex intervention. The guidance for complex interventions produced by the UK's Medical Research Council (MRC) [57,58] acknowledges that randomized controlled trials are not always feasible or appropriate, whilst retaining a preference for experimental design. It is also highly committed to "outcome evaluation"; regarding "process evaluation" as useful but not an alternative to outcome evaluation. Although it avoids a rigid commitment to experimental models, the MRC guidance does not fully address the problems of multiple causality and the time lag between discovery research and new therapies being adopted. The MRC message for evaluating TMR as a complex intervention is to *measure outcomes if at all possible*.

An alternative model that does not depend so much on outcomes is the "use and transformation model" [59]. This model is premised on the belief that measuring outcomes often understates the full benefits of research. It challenges the underlying philosophy of the "outcomes approach" that if information from research is not used it has no value and does not become part of the stock of knowledge. Traditional bibliometric analysis of publications, citations, and patents does not take into account other important users of research findings, such as policy makers, campaigners, and patients. Corley proposes that "knowledge value communities," i.e. all the users of particular pieces or areas of research, should be identified; and repeated uses of research findings, breadth of uses, and the ability to create new uses should be measured and evaluated. The problem with this model is that the investment in data collection for the evaluation would be considerable and would risk becoming disproportionate to the initial research investment.

There are some similarities between the "use and transformation" model and what is known as the "payback approach." The latter attempts to identify knowledge production, research targeting, and capacity building; informing policies and product development; health and health sector benefits; and the broader economic and social benefits in its evaluative criteria. It is not always possible in practice to obtain all of the necessary information, so selective information may often be collected, such as numbers of publications and presentations and assessments of existing and potential impact on policy and behavior [60].

Another good example of how a research program can be evaluated is the conceptual framework developed for clinical trial networks in the United States [45]. This participatory approach to evaluation was adopted because the network had multiple goals and its participating stakeholders had different agendas and priorities. Unless all were involved in developing the framework, it is unlikely that any emerging evaluation conclusions would have been shared. Stakeholders were asked to complete the sentence; "coordinated clinical research networks will be successful if...", in order for evaluators to then develop a framework of success factors. This approach was used by the author for his interviews with funders and practitioners. Answers were noted and used to create clusters or conceptual headings that could be incorporated in the basic program logic model and its evaluation.

Three key themes emerged from the interviews with TMR funders and practitioners. The first theme was outcomes. There was considerable agreement that TMR should ultimately have tangible benefits or outcomes; ranging from the modestly specific to macro level economic benefits. These included

- Goals beyond discovery, such as clinical trials
- New treatment options
- Improved patient benefits
- Improved health
- Speeding up drug development
- Economic benefits either for pharmaceutical companies or national economies

Surprisingly, there were only three answers clustered into the second theme, which was about process. These included

- Knowledge about how to run successful research teams
- New skills to link basic science to health care more quickly
- Creative ideas are brought to bear on unsolved problems

The third theme was centred on attitudes and understanding. Answers included

- Realistic expectation about what can be achieved from TMR
- Subsequent assessment needs to take into account confounding factors and externalities
- Feasible targets
- For evaluation, one size will not fit all
- TMR goals are more than discovery science
- Funders are better able to understand the merits of TMR proposals
- Applicants understand the push factors from basic science and the pull factors from clinical science
- Applicants understand where their proposals contribute along the development trajectory

The final part of the evaluation model was developed from an assessment of Scottish health priorities, as well as mortality and morbidity data. This assessment revealed that there are broad categories of disease that contribute significantly to people in Scotland having lower life expectancy compared to the rest of the UK. There are also important differences between the diseases that contribute most to mortality and morbidity. The Scottish evaluation dimension was obtained from answers to questions about the potential contribution that research studies make towards Scottish health priorities.

Part 1 of the evaluation model asked how the study could be described as translational medicine by reviewing the answers to the "is this TMR?" checklist; and considering how they fit into the stages of the Basic Program Logic Model.

Part 2 sought to assess the value of the study through the following questions.

1. Is there any direct contribution to high-level outcomes such as
    - New treatments
    - Improved patient benefits
    - Improved health
    - Accelerated drug development
    - Economic benefits
2. Are there other specific outcomes such as
    - Goals beyond discovery, such as clinical trials
    - Improved diagnosis
    - New biomarkers
    - Other
3. Has the study informed the process of TMR and the way it might be done in the future?
4. Have the results/findings from the study been used?
5. If so, by whom?
6. Have the results led to further research?
7. Has there been any impact on policy or behavior?
8. Will the study help change attitudes to, and understanding of, TMR?

Part 3 sought to capture the Scottish dimension through the answers to the questions about the TMR study's contribution to Scottish health priorities.

The major omission from the model is that it does not attempt to measure acceleration in drug development. This was partly due to the short timescale available for the project, and also because high attrition rates [61] and the lack of translational results available [39] make it difficult to find data that represent a scientifically fair comparison between the 14 CSO studies and medical research more generally.

5.6 Piloting the Evaluation Model

The first and most obvious feature from the pattern of answers to these questions was that all of the studies could be described as encompassing basic research, but only 57% included clinical research. There was a conceptual link between basic and clinical research in 71% of the studies. However, this is not sufficient to make a decision about whether the research should be described as TMR. This only becomes possible if it can be demonstrated from answers to the questions about increased understanding, benefits, and contributions to TMR methods/techniques. Twenty-nine percent of the studies were either basic or clinical research with no immediately apparent TMR features. Thirty-six percent of the studies had increased understanding of the pathology of disease, the operating system for a new therapy, or safety/toxicity. Fourteen percent of the studies had identified a potential benefit for patients. Twenty-one percent of the studies contributed to biomarker development. There was some overlap in the preceding figures. Finally, 21% of the studies made a contribution to a new technique or methodological improvement. This figure was in addition to the 36% of studies that had contributed to increased understanding of disease pathology, operating system for new therapy, or safety/toxicity. Taking these two figures together, 57% of the studies were found to have a translational outcome that went beyond either basic or clinical research.

None of the selected studies covered more than one step in the "translational journey," although one project both looked forward to application and fed backwards into better understanding of pathology and/or mode of action. Given the limited amount of funding (approximately $50,000 per study), and the expectation to complete within a year, this is not perhaps surprising.

The second set of questions was designed to gather information about outcomes; that is how TMR is carried out and general attitudes towards translation. The question — "does the study look forward to application and feed backwards into understanding of pathology and/or mode of action?" — was intended to be an ambitious test of the dual bench-to-bedside and bedside-to-bench philosophy. One study easily passed this test. The investigation of natural antibiotic production in the female reproductive tract could potentially lead to less invasive diagnosis of ectopic pregnancy and add to knowledge about natural antibiotics in the fallopian tubes and the womb [62]. A second study could be said to have been forward-looking in terms of improved design, conduct, and reporting of animal studies, whilst also looking backwards in the translational process by providing a possible explanation why reliance on the results of animal studies had not led to successful clinical trials in humans [63], even though the study did not involve direct basic or clinical research.

This initial analysis suggests that 36% of the studies seemed to be basic or clinical research rather than TMR. One study that could be described as basic research was the investigation of proinflammatory cytokines as possible biomarkers for stroke [64]. Three novel biomarkers were measured in two groups of older people; one where subjects later had an ischemic stroke and the other where they did not have a stroke. Of the three potential biomarkers, adiponectin at reduced levels was found to be associated with the risk of having an ischemic stroke and was also associated with increased inflammation. No differences were found for the two other potential biomarkers. The researchers concluded by proposing further research to confirm their initial finding. Although this study has potential for future TMR (examining the benefit of a therapy that increases the level of adiponectin, for example), the justification to propose this as an intervention requires more supporting evidence.

The questions that sought to assess the value of the CSO TMR grants were designed to identify if there were any useful study outputs. No attempt was made to quantify the value of the outputs.

There were four high-level outcomes. Two were for improved patient benefits (the finding that the new HPV vaccine should also provide protection against some non-cervical cancers and the ability to identify in advance patients who would become resistant to corticosteroid treatment) and two were for potential economic benefits. Other specific outcomes included data about HPV types in Scotland which would be a base line for future prevalence studies after the introduction of the new vaccine; a new biomarker that could be used for a less invasive method of diagnosing ectopic pregnancy; and new techniques including a validated proteomic technology for brain tumours and a new technology for analysing chromatid levels in metaphase cells.

One study — a systematic literature review — has informed the way TMR should be done in the future through the publication of an international statement of Good Laboratory Practice for the use of animal stroke models. Five other studies have had their findings used in a number of different ways; three as a basis for more research, one as an application to carry out a clinical trial, and the Scottish data collected was used for the promotion of the new HPV vaccine and a symposium for small vessel translational research was held. In most cases, the findings of these studies have been used by other researchers; the exception being public health. This model eschewed counting the number of resulting publications or citations, preferring instead to try and grasp how the findings have been used. This further research has included more glioma proteomic work ($1.5 million funding attracted), assessment of small vessel changes in the Stroke-Prone Spontaneously Hypertensive rat model, and a test of clinical application.

These high-level outcomes (4), other specific outcomes (5), and the use of findings (5), including the statement of Good Laboratory Practice for the use of animal stroke models, are evidence that these studies generated some clear translational outcomes. Ten of the studies generated these outcomes (71% generated some form of translational outcome, whereas 29% did not). The outcome analysis suggests a slightly higher figure for translational research than the initial analysis from the "is this TMR?" question. It is a matter of judgement whether these outcomes represent good value for the funders of these studies. Ideally, there should be some standardized method for measuring value. This model does not do this, although some studies could have a financial value attached to the funding for further research. One of the outputs was negative, when it was discovered that multidrug resistance proteins efflux transporters were not contributing to tyrosine kinase inhibitor insensitivity in chronic myeloid leukaemia. It is theoretically possible that this finding has saved wasted expenditure on future research in this area, but there is no obvious way of measuring this saving. Although it is disappointing to have negative findings, which may mean there is no "immediate translation," by adding to the body of accumulated knowledge it may influence the design of future basic or clinical science which subsequently go on to be translational.

The final feature of the evaluation model takes into account the prevalence, incidence, and morbidity of disease in Scotland

and the health priorities of the Scottish Government [65,66]. Of the 14 studies, 64% had the aim of increasing life expectancy, 21% aimed to improve the management of long-term conditions, and 7% aimed to make health care safer. The answers to the Scottish dimension questions show that 93% of the studies are aligned with Scottish health priorities. The alignment will also be relevant to other countries with a similar disease-burden [17] and where long-term conditions are becoming increasingly significant [67]. These questions also suggest that it possible to use national or international data such as that collected by WHO [68,67] for evaluations of TMR that reflect individual country's health priorities.

The root definitions of TMR provided earlier in this chapter are examples that help us understand TMR as a system linking stages of research. The "choices framework" (which is represented later in Fig. 5.3) implies that TMR as a system, as research stages, and as research processes are mutually exclusive. However, this is not the approach adopted by this evaluation model. Instead, the new broad definition of TMR as an interdependent chain includes both research stages and processes as part of the TMR system. The sets of questions that are linked by the Basic Program Logic Model are used to create a picture for various TMR studies that have been funded through a particular program, as well as a more specific picture for individual projects. The answers provide information in a structured way, which allows general comparisons to be made between studies and more considered judgements to be made of individual projects. It may not be possible to answer all of the questions, in which case the picture of TMR may be limited to the stage or process under investigation.

In summary, the evaluation model has shown that 64% of the CSO studies were initially assessed as having some features of translational research. This figure rose to 71% when the outputs/outcomes of the studies were examined. It would be interesting to assess the impact and value of these outcomes. This would require both a longer period of time to have elapsed between the completion of the studies and their assessment, and an agreed method of measuring value. As has been shown by the *Medical Research: What's It Worth?* report [7], this would become a major research enterprise. However, the model has shown that it is possible to collect data that can be used to provide an initial evaluation of whether a study should be described as translational, identify its early translational outputs and outcomes, and assess its relevance to Scottish health priorities.

This study has largely depended on the author's judgement, whether it was in selecting articles from the literature review, identifying the definitions of TMR, assessing the Chief Scientist Office translational medicine research studies, to reviewing Scottish health priorities and mortality and morbidity data. There was always the risk of subjective bias. However, this was partially mitigated by the additional interview data and the extensive literature review. The subjectivity risk could be further mitigated in future evaluation studies by providing more detailed criteria for assessing the answers to questions, and introducing more extensive consultation and assessment by selected stakeholders of critical judgements such as the new broader definition of TMR, which this study uses, or the checklist assessments for the research reports.

Ideally, the TMR studies used to pilot the evaluation model would have been taken from more than one funding source, and they would also have had greater variation in size and length of time of operation. In the absence of a common data base for TMR, it is difficult to envisage how it would be possible to identify a representative sample of studies. There were clear advantages in using the Chief Scientist Office TMR studies. The number was manageable for this small study; final reports were available in a common format, which aided comparative analysis; and it was possible to use the model to evaluate individual research studies and also the funding program itself.

5.7 Additional Comment on Definitions

The comparison of the definitions and descriptions of TMR that can be found in the selected core papers and the interviews demonstrate that there are differences of emphasis or focus that depend on the scale and scope of TMR under consideration. Descriptions that placed TMR in the wider context of the organization of medical research were more likely also to be concerned about the structure of university medical research, career pathways, and public and private sector collaboration [53]. Descriptions that focused on the day-to-day difficulties of conducting TMR were more likely to give attention to the technical problems of developing suitable biomarkers or the bioinformatics required to analyze the vast amount of information being generated [51]. This confirmed the need to be clear about having an agreed definition of TMR prior to deciding how TMR should be evaluated.

The stages in developing a new working definition also reflect different ways of thinking about TMR, from "a purposeful drug development process" through "a broader perspective than drug development," to "an interdependent chain," which includes biomarker development, streamlining clinical trials, and bioinformatics.

Perhaps the most important difference in the definitions was whether or not TMR stops at approval for use of a new drug or therapy [3]. The second gap in translation, bringing the new therapy into use for those who would benefit from it [69], takes the definition of TMR beyond applied molecular science and therapy development into the organization of healthcare and policy implementation. Woolf has argued that overcoming this second gap in translation is as important as the first. It is likely to benefit more people and is therefore economically essential [70]. In so far as definitions of TMR are compared, rather than just stated in the literature, it is this difference that is the most likely to be mentioned [71,72].

The first step in developing an evaluation model for TMR is to decide how it should be defined. In particular, should it be defined as a system and where should we draw its boundaries. A second step, to be "pragmatic and proportional" [73], is to decide whether the focus should be on the stage (or stages) or process (or processes) of TMR and, if so, which ones?

These choices may be represented in a choices framework (Fig. 5.3).

These choices for the evaluation of TMR depend, *inter alia*, on the reasons for undertaking the evaluation, the commissioner of the evaluation's interest in TMR, and the timescale (both for the evaluation to be carried out and for how long after the TMR was funded consequences/outcomes be sought). Although the choices framework will not lead in itself to consistency in how TMR is

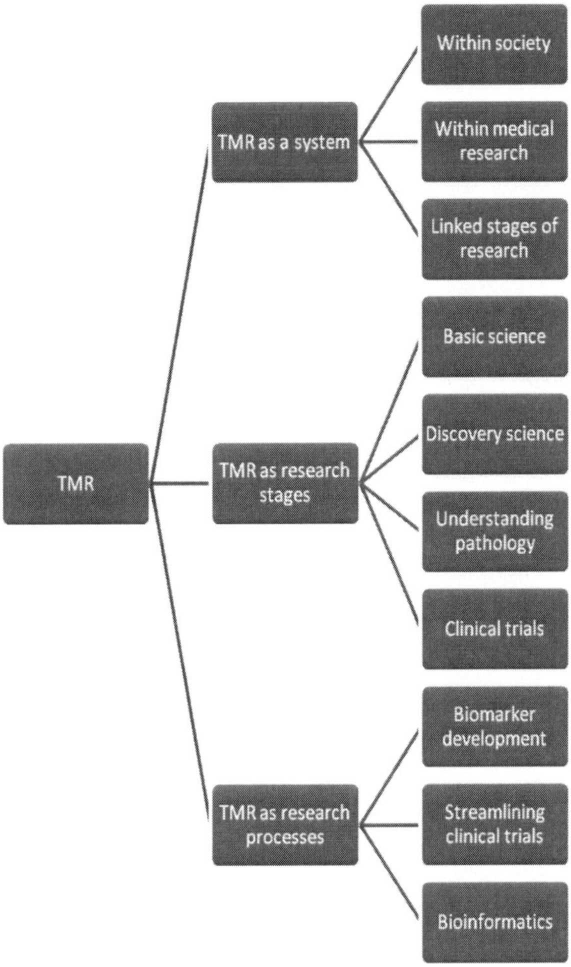

Figure 5.3 Choices framework for the evaluation of TMR.

evaluated, it should lead to clarity about what is being evaluated and reduce the risk of over generalized conclusions.

5.8 Implications for Future Evaluation of TMR

This study, notwithstanding its limitations, has shown that it is possible to develop an evaluation model and demonstrated how it might be used to evaluate TMR. Future evaluations could learn from the experience of creating the "interdependent chain" definition of TMR and the subsequent evaluation model. In conclusion, I propose the following key recommendations for future evaluation of TMR. First, a wider range of TMR research should be evaluated, including larger pieces of research and research from different funding agencies. Second, future evaluations need to be clear about how they define translational research and whether they are attempting a pragmatic evaluation with clearly determined boundaries, or a more ambitious evaluation of TMR as a wider system. Third, consideration should be given to consulting key stakeholders about the definition of TMR being used and the criteria for judgements that affect the evaluation outcomes. Finally, TMR should be subject to more analytical evaluation, which seeks not only to assess the longer term impact but also to distinguish its impact from the consequences of structural changes within the pharmaceutical industry and academia.

References

1. Medical Research Council (2008). Developing and evaluating complex interventions: new guidance. *London: Medical Research Council.*
2. Wellcome Trust (2009). *Wellcome Trust Awards* (Online). www.wellcome.ac.uk/Funding/Technology-transfer/Awards/index.htm. (Accessed 18 October 2009).
3. Albani, S. and Prakken, B. (2009). The advancement of translational medicine-from regional challenges to global solutions. *Nature Medicine*, **15**, pp. 1006–1009.
4. Wehling, M. (2008). Translational medicine: science or wishful thinking? *Journal of Translational Medicine*, **6**, pp. 31, doi:10.1186/1479-5876-6-31.
5. Aronson, J. K., Cohen, A., and Lewis, L. D. (2008). Clinical pharmacology–providing tools and expertise for translational medicine. *British Journal of Clinical Pharmacology*, **65**, pp. 154–157.
6. UK Evaluation Forum (2006). Medical research: assessing the benefits to society. *London: The Academy of Medical Sciences, Medical Research Council and Wellcome Trust.*

7. Health Economics Research Group, Office Of Health Economics, Rand Europe (2008). Medical research: What's it worth? Estimating the economic benefits from medical research in the UK. *London: Wellcome Trust/MRC/The Academy of Medical Sciences.*
8. Hughes, B. (2010). 2009 FDA drug approvals. *Nature Reviews Drug Discovery*, **9**, pp. 89–92.
9. Mitchell, P. (2008). Investor malaise stalks UK, European biotech. *Nature Biotechnology*, **26**, pp. 256–257.
10. Mitchell, P. (2009). Venture capital shifts strategies, startups suffer. *Nature Biotechnology*, **27**, pp. 103–104.
11. Paul, S.M., Dunwiddie, C.T., Lindborg, S.R., Munos, B.H., Mytelka, D.S., Persinger, C.C., and Schacht, A.L. (2010). How to improve R&D productivity: the pharmaceutical industry's grand challenge. *Nature Reviews Drug Discovery*, **9**, pp. 203–214.
12. Dimasi, J.A. and Grabowski, H.G. (2007). The cost of biopharmaceutical R&D: is biotech different? *Managerial and Decision Economics*, **28**, pp. 469–479.
13. Mittra, J. (2007). Life science innovation and the restructuring of the pharmaceutical industry: merger, aquisition and strategic alliance behaviour of large firms. *Technology Analysis and Strategic Management*, **19** (3), pp. 279–301.
14. Walker, J. (2010). M&A activity in 2009. *Nature Reviews Drug Discovery*, **9**, pp. 95.
15. Czerepak, E.A. and Ryser, S. (2008). Drug approvals and failures: implications for alliances. *Nature Reviews Drug Discovery*, **7**, pp. 197–198.
16. Tralau-Stewart, C.J., Ayed, A., Kleyn, D.E., and Wyatt, C.A. (2009). Drug discovery: new models for industry-academic partnerships. *Drug Discovery Today*, **14**, pp. 95–101.
17. Sutherland, K. and Coyle, N. (2009). Quality in healthcare in England, Wales, Scotland and Northern Ireland, *London, The Health Foundation.*
18. Green, S. and Miles, R. (2007). The burden of disease and illness in the UK: a preliminary assessment to inform the development of UK health research and development priorities. *Oxford Healthcare Associates.*
19. Harvard School of Public Health (1996). The Global Burden of Disease: a comprehensive assessment of mortality and disability from diseases and injuries and risk factors in 1990 and projected to 2020. *Harvard University Press.*

20. Cairns, J. (2006). Providing guidance to the NHS: the Scottish Medicines Consortium and the National Institute for Clinical Excellence compared. *Health Policy*, **76**, pp. 134–143.
21. Faden, L.B. and Kaitin, K.I. (2008). Assessing the performance of EMEA's centralised procedure: a comparative analysis with the USA FDA. *Drug Information Journal*, **42**, pp. 45–55.
22. Longstaff, C., Grey, E., Stebbings, R., and Whitton, C.M. (2009). How do we assure the quality of biological medicines? *Drug Discovery Today*, **14**, pp. 50–54.
23. Tufts Center for the Study of Drug Development (2010). Rising protocol complexity, execution burden varies widely by phase and TA. *May/June Tufts CSDD Impact report. Boston:* (Tufts Center for the Study of Drug Development).
24. Woolf, S.H. (2008). The meaning of translational research and why it matters. *Journal of the American Medical Association*, **299**, pp. 211–213.
25. Dougherty, E.R. (2009). Translational science: epistemology and the investigative process. *Current Genomics*, **10**, pp. 102–109.
26. Pincus, H.A. (2009). Challenges and pathways for clinical and translational research: why is this research different from all other research? *Academic Medicine*, **84**, pp. 411–412.
27. Chief scientist office (2006). Experimental medicine-translational medicine research grants. *Biomedical and Therapeutic Research Committee*, (Chief Scientist Office, Scottish Executive).
28. Saijo, N. (2002). Translational study in cancer research. *Internal Medicine*, **41**, pp. 770–773.
29. Niederhuber, J.E. (2010). Translating discovery to patient care. *JAMA*, **303**, pp. 1088–1089.
30. Fontanarosa, P.B. and Deangelis, C.D. (2003). Translational medical research. *JAMA*, **289**, pp. 2133, doi:10.1001/jama.289.16.
31. Littman, B.H., Di Mario, L., Plebani, M., and Marincola, F.M. (2007). What's next in translational medicine? *Clinical Science*, **112**, pp. 217–227.
32. Pardridge, W.M. (2003). Translational science: what is it and why is it so important? *Drug Discovery Today*, **8**, pp. 813–815.
33. Goldblatt, E.M. and Lee, W.H. (2010). From bench to bedside: the growing use of translational research in cancer medicine. *American Journal of Translational Research*, **2**, pp. 1–18.

34. Horig, H. and Pullman, W. (2004). From bench to clinic and back: perspective on the 1st IQPC Translational Research conference. *Journal of Translational Research*, 2 (44), doi:10.1186/1479-5876.

35. Chan, J.Y.H., Chan, S.H.H., and Chang, A.Y.W. (2005). New insights on brain stem death: from bedside to bench. *Progress in Neurobiology*, **77**, pp. 396–425.

36. Rubio, D.M., Anderson, K.E., Baez, A., Esposito, K,. Lee, L.S., Marantz, P.R., Platt, L.D., Schoenbaum, E.E., and Schteingart, D.E. (2010). Defining translational research: implications for training. *Academic Medicine*, **85**, pp. 470–475.

37. Van Den Hoonaard, D.K. (2009). Moving toward a three-way intersection in translational research: a sociological perspective. *Qualitative Health Research*, **19**, pp. 1783–1787.

38. Milne, C.-P. and Kaitin, K.I. (2009). Translational medicine: an engine of change for bringing new technology to community health. *Science Translational Medicine*, **1** (5), DOI:10.1126/scitranslmed.3000222.

39. Heller, C. and De Melo-Martin, I. (2009). Clinical and translational science awards: can they increase the efficency and speed of clinical and translational research? *Academic Medicine*, **84**, pp.424–432.

40. Fiscella, K., Bennett, N.M., and Szilagyi, P.G. (2008). Nomenclature in translational research. *JAMA*, **299**, pp. 2148–2149; author reply pp. 2149–2150.

41. Graham, I.D. and Tetroe, J. (2008). Nomenclature in translational research. *JAMA*, **299**, pp. 2149; author reply pp. 2149–2150.

42. Rutter, M. and Plomin, R. (2009). Pathways from science findings to health benefits. *Psychological Medicine*, **39**, pp. 529–542.

43. Checkland, P. (1999). *Systems thinking, systems practice*, (Chichester, John Wiley and Sons Ltd.)

44. Checkland, P. and Winter, M. (2006). Process and content: two ways of using SSM. *Journal of the Operational Research Society*, **57**, pp. 1435–1441.

45. Kagan, J.M., Kane, M., Quinlan, Kathleen M, Rosas, S., and Trochim, W.M. (2009). Developing a conceptual framework for an evaluation system for the NIAID HIV/AIDS clinical trials networks. *Health Research Policy Systems*, **7** (12), doi:10.1186/1478-4505-7-12.

46. Centers for disease control (2005). Introduction to Program Evaluation for Public Health Programs: A self-study guide.

47. Sung, N.S., Catanese, V., Crowley, W.F., Jr., Dobs, A., Genel, M., Getz, K., Grebb, J., Johnson, S.B., Korn, A., Larson, E.L., Martinez, R.A., Reece, E.A., Rimoin, D., Salber, P., Sandy, L., Scheinberg, D., Sherwood, L.M., Slavkin, H., and Tilson, H. (2003). Central challenges facing the national clinical research enterprise. *JAMA*, **289**, pp. 1278–1287.
48. Fitzgerald, G.A. (2005). Opinion: anticipating change in drug development: the emerging era of translational medicine and therapeutics. *Nature Reviews, Drug Discovery.* **4**, pp. 815–818.
49. Marincola, F.M. (2003). Translational medicine: a two-way road. *Journal of Translational Medicine*, **1**, doi:10.1186/1479-5876-1-1.
50. Lee, W.-H. (2009). Translational medical research: present and future. *American Journal of Translational Research*, **1**, pp. 99–100.
51. Webb, C.P. and Pass, H.I. (2004). Translation research: from accurate diagnosis to appropriate treatment. *Journal of Translational Medicine*, **2** (35), doi:10.1186/1479-5876-2-35.
52. Littman, B.H., Di Mario, L., Marincola, F.M., and Plebani, M. (2007). What's next in translational medicine? *Clinical Science*, **112**, pp. 217–227.
53. Zerhouni, E.A. (2005). Translational and clinical science - time for a new vision. *New England Journal of Medicine*, 353, 1621–1623.
54. Mankoff, S., Brander, C., Ferrone, S., and Marincola, F.M. (2004). Lost in Translation: bbstacles to translational medicine. *Journal of Translational Medicine*, **2** (14), doi:10.1186/1479-5876-2-14.
55. FDA. (2006). *Critical path opportunities report*, (US Department of Health and Human Services, March, 2006).
56. Nussenblatt, R.B., Marincola, F.M., and Schechter, A.N. (2010). Translational medicine - doing it backwards. *Journal of Translational Medicine*, **8** (12).
57. Craig, P., Dieppe, P., Macintyre, S., Mitchie, S., Nazareth, I., and Petticrew, M. (2008). Developing and evaluating complex interventions: the new Medical Research Guidance. *British Medical Journal*, **337**, pp. 979–983.
58. Medical Research Council. (2008). *Update on translation research* (Online). www.mrc.ac.uk/Opportunities/index.htm. (Accessed 31 October 2008).
59. Corley, E.A. (2007). A use-and-transformation model for evaluating public R&D: illustrations from polycystic ovarian syndrome (PCOS) research. *Evaluation and Program Planning*, **30**, pp. 21–35.

60. Raftery, J., Buxton, M., Green, C., and Hanney, S. (2009). Assessing the impact of England's National Health Service R&D Health Technology Assessment Program using the 'payback' approach. *International Journal of Technology Assessment in Health Care*, **25**, pp. 1–5.
61. O'connell, D. and Roblin, D. (2006). Translational research in the pharmaceutical industry: from bench to bedside. *Drug Discovery Today*, **11**, pp. 833–838.
62. Horne, A., Cameron, S., Critchley, H., and King, A. (2008). Effects of chlamydia on natural antibiotic production in the female reproductive tract - could altered antibiotic production be exploited as a test for ectopic pregnancy? *Focus on Research.* (Edinburgh: Chief Scientist Office, Scottish Executive Health Department).
63. Macleod, M., Kelly, P., Sandercock, P., Sena, E., Vesterinen, H., and Williams, C. (c.2008). Improving the design, conduct and reporting of animal studies in experimental stroke. *Focus on Research.* (Edinburgh: Chief Scientist Office, Scottish Executive Health Department).
64. Stott, D.J., Ford, I., Lowe, G.D.O., and Satter, N. (c.2008). Proinflamatory cytokines as biomarkers for risk of stroke. *Focus on Research.* (Edinburgh: Chief Scientist Office, Scottish Executive Health Department).
65. Scottish Government (2007). Better health, better care: action plan. (Edinburgh: Scottish Government).
66. Scottish Government (2009). Improving health and wellbeing of people with long term health conditions in Scotland: a national action plan. (Edinburgh: Scottish Government).
67. World Health Organisation. (2008). 2008–2013 *Action Plan for the Global Strategy for the Prevention and Control of Noncommunicable Diseases* (Online). (World Health Organisation) www.whqlibdoc.who.int/publications/2009/9789241597418_eng.pdf. (Accessed 6 May 2010).
68. World Health Organisation (2004). The Global Burden of Disease: 2004 Update. (World Health Organisation).
69. Cooksey, D. (2006). A Review of UK Health Research Funding. www.hm-treasury.gov.uk/independent_reviews/cooksey_review/cookseyreview_index.cfm.
70. Woolf, S.H. (2007). Potential health and economic consequences of misplaced priorities. *Journal of the American Medical Association*, **297**, pp. 523–526. Doi : 10.1001/jama.

71. Dougherty, D. and Conway, P.H. (2008). The "3T's" road map to transform US health care: the how of high-quality care. *Journal of the American Medical Association*, **299**, pp. 2319–2321.
72. Sonntag, K.-C. (2005). Implementation of translational medicine. *Journal of Translational Medicine*, **3** (33), doi:10.1186/1479-5876-3-33.
73. Allen, L. (2010). The art of evaluating the impact of medical science. *Bulletin of the World Health Organisation*, **88**, pp. 4, doi: 10.2471/BLT.09.074823.

Part 3

State-of-the-Art in the Science and Technology

Chapter 6

Emerging Concepts in Biomarker Discovery: Cancer Immunotherapy and Degenerative Disease of the Eye as Model Systems

Robert B. Nussenblatt[a,*] and Francesco M. Marincola[b]

[a] *National Eye Institute, NIH,*
10 Center Drive Bethesda, Maryland 20892, USA
[b] *Trans-NIH Center for Human Immunology, National Institutes of Health Director, CC/CHI FOCIS Center of Excellence, Bethesda, Maryland 20892, USA*
*nussenblattr@nei.nih.gov

6.1 Introduction

In this chapter, we define translational medicine as a coordinated attempt to enhance the efficacy of discovery in the biomedical field by improving stakeholder interactions [1,2]. Among the various hurdles that hamper the achievement of this goal, we have identified the limited knowledge of human pathophysiology compared to the wealth of basic information on fundamental biological processes as a major challenge. Although we have a strong grasp on how cells live, communicate, travel, and die in a hypothetical organism, very

Translational Medicine: The Future of Therapy
Edited by James Mittra and Christopher-Paul Milne

ISBN 978-981-4316-99-6 (Hardback), 978-981-4364-84-3 (eBook)
www.panstanford.com

little is known about how they participate in the process of life when disease strikes. In particular, little information is available about how basic biological processes behave across the genetic variability of humans and their diseases or how the environment may influence such behavior in ways that may not be suspected by studying simplified experimental models in the sterility of the laboratory. Thus, we have argued [3,4], and continue to do so [5], that translational medicine is a two-way process with a bedside-to-bench component that has not been sufficiently appreciated in the past. Among the benefits of an approach that emphasizes direct clinical observation for an accurate understanding of human pathophysiology is the potential to identify indicators of disease status that are peculiar to a given patient and may help the decision-making process that guides selection and treatment options.

In this chapter, we argue that these indicators or biomarkers are more likely to be identified if human samples are studied at the appropriate time points, relevant tissues are selected, and modern high-throughput approaches are used. In particular, we discuss how this approach was applied to improve understanding of complex problems, such as the treatment of cancer with biological manipulation and the biology of degenerative disease of the eye. We hope that such examples will illustrate the usefulness of studying humans directly through discovery-driven, hypothesis generating approaches. To push the argument even further, we suggest that direct observation of human disease may provide new insights about the natural history of disease and its reaction to treatment in specific circumstances. Alternative mechanisms, which are conceivable given our basic understanding of biology, we argue simply do not apply to human reality. We refer to the observational approach as "facts-driven research." By facts, we mean occurrences that are unarguably linked to the determinism of a given pathophysiological condition that affects human beings. Facts-driven research is presented in antithesis to hypotheses derived from observation in experimental models, which may or may not apply to human reality.

6.2 What Is a Biomarker?

A biomarker is an objectively measurable indicator of a biological state, pathogenic process, or pharmacologic response to a therapeutic intervention. A PubMed search for articles containing the term "biomarker(s)" in their title yielded 12,451 hits by August 10, 2010. This emphasizes the eagerness among researchers to identify parameters of relevance to clinical decision making. Indeed, most health care spending in the United States is directed at the treatment of chronic diseases like degenerative neurologic disorders, cardiovascular insufficiency, and cancer [6,7]. Due to the protracted nature of these conditions, it is difficult to efficiently judge the long-term benefit of new treatments so predictors of clinical utility become critical for early decision making in drug development [8]. Biomarkers can (1) guide patient selection and stratification for the most appropriate treatment; (2) identify most suitable targets of therapy; (3) measure treatment effect; (4) verify hypothesized mechanisms of drug action and/or identify novel unsuspected ones; (5) assess and categorize disease status or disease burden; and (6) represent surrogate early markers of long-term treatment benefit. Moreover, biomarkers as prognostic indicators can aid decisions about when to begin treatment [9]. For example, identifying biological characteristics related to the genetic background of the patient or their disease before treatment could be used to stratify patients according to their likelihood of response to targeted therapies. Identification of early biological changes in response to therapy that could be linked to lengthening of survival or improved quality of life (surrogate biomarkers) could improve the effectiveness of clinical trials and facilitate early decisions about the effectiveness of a given treatment. This is particularly useful in the case of chronic diseases for which benefits can only be assessed after years or even decades.

A special note should be made concerning biological biomarkers. It is logical during the monitoring of a clinical trial to identify whether the drug being tested is inducing the experimentally predicted biological effect. Obviously, if for various reasons related to the pharmacokinetics or the pharmacodynamics of the drug, or other unpredicted circumstances, the treatment does not achieve the biological effect that it was supposed to produce, the interpretation of a clinically unfavorable result will be quite different than if the biological end point had been achieved. We prefer, however, a broader view of these monitoring efforts and prefer to use the term "mechanistic" biomarkers that can identify, using high-throughput technology, not only expected biological effects but also novel and unexpected ones (an example is given later when discussing the analysis of the mechanism of action of interleukin-2 for the treatment of advanced cancer). Thus, various kinds of biomarkers are critical for the selection and assessment of treatment both in the research setting and in clinical practice. Specific examples are given throughout this chapter.

While in the past biomarkers were predominantly based on morphological aspects of pathological specimens, in the last few years the portfolio has broadened to include other aspects of biomedical investigation including, in particular, molecular testing. A number of good examples are emerging. Mutations in B-RAF and c-KIT genes guide the selection of patients with melanoma likely to respond to treatment with the respective pathway inhibitor [10]. Early decrease in viral load in response to anti-viral therapy represents a powerful indicator of long-term survival of patients with human immune deficiency virus (HIV) infection [11,12] and it is now used to assess other biological parameters as a surrogate of disease progression [13]. Rapid recurrence of viral detection after first line treatment of hepatitis C virus (HCV) infection is an early indicator of future treatment failure and it is used in deciding whether to continue a poorly tolerated therapy [14]. Broad genome-wide studies of HCV infection recently yielded independent validation that polymorphisms in interferon (IFN)-λ region are associated with the natural history of the disease and its responsiveness to IFN-α therapy [15,16]. We have long searched for mechanistic biomarkers to test whether a given treatment achieved its biological end point: does active-specific immunization with cancer antigens enhance the frequency of cancer-recognizing T cells [17]? We have also been interested in characterizing the mechanisms of action of anti-cancer agents within the tumor microenvironment when such mechanisms were unknown: what are the intra-tumoral effects of the systemic administration of high-dose interleukin (IL)-2 [18] or the local administration of Toll-like receptor (TLR) agonists [19]? These kind of investigations help us to select among several hypotheses those that actually occur in clinical conditions. For example, it was believed that the predominant effect of systemic IL-2 administration was an increase in capillary leak syndrome, which enhanced the homing of tumor-recognizing lymphocytes at the tumor site. Transcriptional profiling of melanoma metastases undergoing IL-2 therapy ruled out this mechanism and clearly demonstrated that IL-2 acts instead by inducing a cytokine storm which eventually leads to the pro-inflammatory activation of tumor infiltrating macrophages; these in turn start the activation of pro-inflammatory mechanisms in the target tissue [18,20,21]. Thus, the search for biomarkers can serve several purposes and success stories are rapidly accumulating [8,9]. Yet, in most cases, the identification of useful biomarkers that could facilitate clinical decision making is still at an early stage.

6.2.1 *The Difficult Path to Biomarker Discovery and Its Relevance to Translational Medicine*

The identification of clinically useful biomarkers has been hampered for a number of reasons [22], but we argue that the foremost impediment is the classic hypothesis-driven model of research, which depends on minimalist experimental animal models for pre-clinical testing and bypasses the study of human disease in its complexity [23]. Although we do not argue that animal-based experimentation has no role to play in the investigation of basic biological principles, we suggest that its current use in the pre-clinical arena is questionable [5]. Translational research should be a two-way process with the bedside-to-bench component providing critical insights for the understanding of human disease [3,4]. It appears that scientists have settled on the more comfortable ground of animal experimentation; regarding this as pristine and easily controllable. This attitude yielded a wealth of conceptual information about biologic phenomena of possible significance, but failed to frame any of them in the context of human disease as recently recognized by a leading experimentalist in the field of immunology [24]. Thus, concepts about potentially important biological processes and, consequently, potentially useful candidate biological markers abound. However, evidence that any of them are relevant to human disease is scant. Publication practices have compounded the problem since most high impact journals strongly favor reiteration of popular work using ever more detailed experimental animal models over the less pristine research performed in humans [25]. The requirements for relevance of experimental work to human pathology is only recently being appreciated and several publishers including traditional scientific organizations begin to recognize the need to expand the breadth of scientific publication [26].

Although there are many hurdles faced by scientists interested in human disease [1,2], we propose that the most significant one faced by those interested in identifying parameters that could guide clinical investigation is the poor design of clinical studies. Most clinical investigations focus on the bench-to-bedside aspects of translational investigations where, if successful, immediate rewards can be expected. In other words, this approach aims to test as quickly as possible concepts arising from experimental approaches for their effectiveness in treating humans. Most of the investigations tend to become less elaborate as they approach the clinical phase, where the aim is to test the largest possible patient population for improvements in survival or, more broadly, curing or mitigating the impact of disease. This approach has failed in the majority of cases because drug design is not based on a direct understanding of human pathophysiology. Furthermore, since no corollary studies are conducted to test whether the treatment reached its biological endpoint in the target tissues, and there is no attempt to understand the cause of failure by studying the tissues, very little is gained by these large and costly studies and the scientific community does not benefit by learning from failure. Bedside-to-bench investigations assume that a clinical trial will not likely succeed and that other investigations should complement the assessment of clinical benefit. This approach, which is aimed at improving our understanding of a disease process, is often disregarded; this less popular direction of translational research requires exhaustive collections of human samples, which is hampered by regulatory concerns and extraordinary costs for storage and sample tracking. Furthermore, it is difficult to publish descriptive analyses in most journals, particularly from studies that yield a negative clinical outcome. Although most recognize the critical role of this approach for the long-term understanding of human pathology, few clinical scientists endorse the application of this principle due to the low probability of short-term reward [23]. Thus, as we have recently suggested [23], the current attitude of the scientific community and the skewed incentives offered to researchers result in

(i) Lack of rigor in selecting hypotheses relevant to human disease to be tested in the laboratory or even later in clinical studies
(ii) Lack of sufficient rigor in conceptualizing clinical studies aimed not only at validation of therapies but also at learning from all results so as to better design subsequent trials

6.2.2 *New Paradigm for Biomarker Discovery: A Global Approach to the Study of Humans*

We propose that if translational research is to be successful, hypothesis-driven research that has dominated the scene during the last century of biomedical investigation should be complemented (not supplanted) by "facts-driven" research. Facts-driven research aims at the identification, among all alternative biological mechanisms that could be hypothesized according to our understanding of biology, only those that actually occur during a given pathophysiological condition. The rationale for this conclusion is based on the simple reasoning that in the presence of hard facts hypotheses are not necessary [4]. On the other hand, when bedside-to-bench investigations cannot provide definitive answers, they may suggest novel hypotheses that can be tested with classical experimental approaches with confidence of their relevance to human disease, because they are based on direct human observation. This paradigm shift was made possible in the last decade by the advent of high-throughput, genome-wide investigations. Before high-throughput technologies came to age, observational and descriptive analyses were not an effective tool to investigate the complexity of human disease and most of the yield derived from observation was due to serendipitous discoveries [27]. With the advent of high-throughput screening, it is now possible to systemically investigate thousands of variables that may affect a clinical condition; increasing the likelihood of successfully identifying relevant information or, in other words, greatly enhancing the chances for serendipity [28,29]. A paradigm shift is brought by the ability to look at biology following a non-linear mathematics approach where patterns are more informative than individual data points [30–34]. Patterns may identify common occurrences within the heterogeneity of humans and their diseases that are necessary for the determinism of a particular phenomenon. We exemplified the usefulness of this approach with the description of the immunologic constant of rejection (ICR) [35]. By applying high-throughput genomics to the study of cancerous tissue undergoing rejection during immunotherapy, we observed recurrent transcriptional patterns during immune-mediated cancer rejection that were independent of treatment or type of cancer [35]. Comparison of our results with others who have applied the same strategy for the study of other aspects of immune-mediated tissue-specific destruction (TSD) such as acute allograft rejection, graft versus host disease, autoimmunity, and acute infection resulting in clearance of the pathogen through destruction of the infected cells; we identified a restricted set of genes that are necessary for the determinism of TSD [36]. Thus, biomarker discovery will likely become a realistic proposition when novel computational approaches applied to the analysis of high-throughput information help scientists identify patterns predictive of clinically relevant events [37]. This paradigm shift does not supplant hypothesis-driven research, rather it should help the selection of hypotheses framed within the reality of human disease; scientists will still need to go back to the bench and test their hypotheses but with better confidence that their work will be relevant [4].

We propose that in the future clinical studies should incorporate a bedside-to-bench strategy in which time and site of collection is forensically chosen and sample, processing, and storage optimized for scientific applications in which high-throughput technologies could be applied for a global approach to the study of humans. In an admittedly oversimplified view, humans, as multi-cellular organisms, are structured according to a hierarchy of genetic interactions that go from genomic DNA, to transcription into RNA and translation into functional units (proteins in different functional statuses) that may or may not differ among cells within a tissue or from different tissues. The study of each layer within this hierarchy provides distinct information. DNA analysis provides information about relatively stable characteristics of cells and tissues that may explain variations among individual patients, or aberrances between normal and abnormal tissues. Messenger RNA (mRNA) informs mostly about the reaction of cells to environmental conditions. We compare transcriptional analysis to the electroencephalographic responses to stimulation which inform us about the reaction to stimulus; thus, while mRNA provides information about the "brain response" of a cell (spikes in response to light), protein analysis provides information about what a cell is doing as the hand covers the eyes when the light is too strong. Since each component provides different types of information and one kind cannot be assumed from the other, clinical research should study humans by evaluating all components simultaneously. Moreover, samples should be obtained at moments relevant to the natural history of a disease or its response to therapy. Since a characteristic of biology is rapid reaction to stimulation, any observations done in steady state conditions (i.e., before a given treatment) may mislead the interpretation of events occurring following a perturbation of the system (i.e., a given treatment). While the technologies will continue to evolve, the important limiting, but non-changing, factor will be the availability of properly collected clinical material to study. In the remaining part of this chapter we discuss how such an approach was applied to the understanding of a complex problem, namely the treatment of cancer with biological manipulation. In the following sections we exemplify how this can be achieved by adopting as models the study of immune responsiveness of melanoma and reviewing the pathophysiology of degenerative disease of the eye. In the former we discuss how high-throughput technology can be used for hypothesis generation, while in the latter, we predominantly focus on the relevance of animal research and the benefits of studying human pathology directly.

6.2.3 *Concepts Emerging from the Study of the Biologic Therapy of Cancer*

The identification of tumor antigens (**TA**) recognized by T cells [38] lead to their utilization as anti-cancer vaccines and provide a powerful tool to analyze in molecular detail the dynamics of developing immune responses in the cancer bearing host [39]. Studies have shown that TA-specific immunization can reliably enhance the frequency circulating tumor-recognizing CD8+ T cells [40] but this enhancement does not correlate with the induction of the desired clinical endpoint: the rejection of cancer [41]. While anti-cancer vaccines come with minimal toxicity but very limited effectiveness, [42,43] treatment with systemic immune stimulators such as IL-2 is associated with significant toxicity. However, IL-2 therapy can induce meaningful cancer regression in about 10% of patients, which is associated with long-term survival [44,45]. It has recently been shown in a randomized clinical trial that the combination of IL-2 and TA vaccination is more effective than either of them alone [46]. This observation helps us understand the requirements for the induction of effective immune responses by focusing on downstream events of TA-specific T cell generation [41,47,48] that could be enhanced by combining systemic immune-stimulation [49]. The identification of predictors of response would greatly enhance the usefulness of this approach, while understanding of the mechanisms leading to activation of vaccine-induced T cells by IL-2 could provide insights useful for the design of next generation agents. Several factors that could affect the relationship between the host and its cancer need to be considered, which can be grouped into two broad categories: variables related to the genetic background of the host and factors related to the genetic heterogeneity of the cancers [50].

Genetic polymorphism may affect immune responsiveness by varying the function of genes associated with antigen presentation, cytokines, killer cell immunoglobulin-like receptors, and leukocyte Fcγ geceptors [51]. Tumor cell biology may affect T cell function through pathways independent of HLA/epitope T cell receptor engagement [47,48]. Several examples of associations between polymorphisms of immune genes and disease outcome, discovered by high-throughput genome wide scanning tools, are emerging from other disciplines. For example, polymorphisms of the interferon (IFN)-λ gene have been shown to play a key role in determining the response of HCV-infected patients to treatment with pegylated IFN-α (an agent also used against several cancers) and ribavarin [15]. Similarly, polymorphisms in the HLA class I region, discovered by high-throughput analysis, predict viral load in patients with HIV [16]. It is possible that the same polymorphisms may explain the different clinical responsiveness of cancer patients to immunotherapy. However, although examples of weak associations have been described for cancer [52,53], no systematic observations of the extent described in other disciplines have been performed to validate these observations [9].

The heterogeneity of cancer is likely to play a key role in determining responsiveness to immunotherapy. The best evidence for this comes from the observation of mixed responses, which are defined as ambiguous behavior of distinct metastases in response to therapy. This is often observed in melanoma; following a cycle of therapy, some metastases melt away while others continue to grow undisturbed [50]. These observations, excluding the genetic background of the host or variations due to treatment as factors determining immune responsiveness, clearly point to subtle genetic differences among autologous tumor masses sufficient to determine distinct phenotypes. Several have looked at somatic factors, identifiable by studying the peripheral circulation of cancer patients, to catch glimpses of distinct cancer biology [9,22]. Screening sera of cancer patients obtained before treatment with systemic IL-2, we tested more than 100 cytokines levels and found that high VEGF levels are a strong predictor of non-responsiveness to therapy. These observations from studying the peripheral circulation stimulated the analysis of cancerous tissue and brought to the conclusion that high VEGF levels in sera correlated to VEGF production by cancer cells [54]. Other potential candidate biomarkers detectable in the peripheral circulations are also being discovered, but no systematic attempt to validate them in large patient cohorts has been conducted.

We have long argued that the direct study of tumors, with the intent of gaining mechanistic insights about tumor immune responsiveness, may be more informative than the study of circulating immune cells of other systemic factors [50,55–58]. The tumor microenvironment, however, is difficult to access in humans and, therefore, immune monitoring has been limited mostly to the study of circulating immune cells that can easily be accessed through venipuncture. Previous observations based on the analysis of cell lines or tissue preparations from excisional biopsies, about which very little clinical information was available, suggested that cutaneous and ocular melanoma segregate into two distinct taxonomies based on global transcript analysis [59]. We proposed that the application of minimally invasive biopsies such as fine needle aspirates (FNA), by leaving the individual metastasis in place, allows for a more direct correlation between biological characteristics studied in the laboratory and the natural or therapy-induced behavior of each lesion [60]. Moreover, by leaving the lesion in place it is possible to perform repeated biopsies that allow for a paired analysis comparing pre-treatment biology with that of the same lesion undergoing [18,19] or following therapy [55]. By prospectively collecting clinical information regarding lesions from which FNA samples had been serially obtained, it was possible to monitor changes in transcriptional programs of individual lesions occurring over time. By adding this temporal dimension to the study of cancer biology, we observed that the two melanoma subgroups did not represent two distinct disease taxonomies but rather two stages of the same rapidly evolving disease [55]. To further evaluate the weight of ontogeny on the molecular sub-classification of cancer, we compared the transcriptional profile of RCC to that of paired normal kidney samples and primary cancers of different histology [61]. This study confirmed that molecular sub-classes result predominantly from the level of differentiation of individual cancers rather than representing distinct taxonomies. When genes expressed by paired normal kidney samples were removed from the analysis, RCC segregated together with cancers of other histology underlying the similarity of the oncogenic process regardless of the tissue origin. Nevertheless, a limited number of RCC-specific genes was identified that might be of relevance to the biological behavior of this disease. These findings emphasize the need to study the relationship between human cancer and its host following a dynamic approach, as changes over time can be significant and rapidly evolve [60].

We applied high-throughput technology to portray transcriptional characteristics unique to metastatic cutaneous melanoma that may be relevant to its immunogenic potential, and identified functional signatures descriptive of immune or other biological functions [62]. Melanoma differentiation antigens (tyrosinase, gp100/PMel17 and MART-1/MelanA) were found to be coordinately expressed, which suggests that their down-regulation or loss of expression during melanoma progression may be related to a central regulatory pathway. This confirms previous studies describing a coordinate loss of expression of MART-1/Melan A and gp100/PMel17 (*SILV*) by melanoma metastases [63–65]. This finding may have important repercussions in the design of TA-specific immunizations or may complicate the interpretation of TA loss variant analysis by broadening loss of expression of TA other than those targeted by a given therapy. More recently, however, we and others have focused on other factors that seem to be stronger predictors of immune responsiveness in cancer. An extensive analysis of melanoma metastases biopsied before treatment, which looked at the expression of the TA targeted by vaccination, ruled this out as a relevant predictor of immune responsiveness [65]; however, genome wide scanning of the same pre-treatment lesions identified immunologic signatures predictive of immune responsiveness [55]. The ability to directly link genetic profiling to clinical history is paramount for future studies. We demonstrated this concept by performing a supervised analysis of lesions undergoing FNA before treatment. Lesions were separated according to their subsequent clinical response to treatment, and transcriptional profiling identified candidate genes predictive of immune responsiveness. These genes were predominantly associated with immune function, suggesting that tumor deposits are pre-conditioned to respond to a tumor microenvironment that is immunologically active even before treatment administration [55]. In particular, the observation that interferon-regulatory factor (IRF)-2 is over-expressed, before treatment, in metastases likely to respond to immunotherapy suggest that tumors are more likely to respond to immunotherapy if they are chronically inflamed in steady state conditions. The inflammatory process may not be sufficient to induce tumor rejection, but it may set the stage for a conversion to an acute inflammatory process during therapy by activation of immune cells present in the tumor tissues [66]. Indeed, a paired analysis of FNA samples obtained before and during therapy underlined this possibility, since lesions that underwent complete response were characterized by the over-expression of IRF-1 following treatment; a counterpart to IRF-2 generally up-regulated during acute inflammation [67]. Interestingly, lesions that did not undergo regression did not demonstrate any significant changes in their transcriptional profile in response to therapy [55]. These findings have been recently confirmed by others in different human cancer systems [9]. Although the underlying reason for the immune activation of some tumors remains to be identified, we recently observed the existence of a subgroup of cancer cells that *in vitro* and *in vivo* display a constitutive activation of endogenous innate immune genes comparable to that of cells infected by a virus (anti-viral state) [68]. Because these changes could be seen both *in vivo* (suggesting that they are not a mere experimental artifact) and *in vitro* in pure cancer cell cultures (suggesting that the anti-viral state is intrinsic to the biology of cancer cells independent of interactions with host cells), we hypothesize that some cancers carry in their own biology the potential to activate immune responses. This phenomenon has been described in other human cancers such as melanoma [48], prostate [69], breast [70], and colorectal cancer [71] and, in some cases, associate with better disease prognosis [9].

While the identification of predictors of responsiveness is important for patient selection and may provide insights about the mechanisms leading to tumor rejection by the host (why are some tumors rejected and some are not?), understanding the mechanisms activated during therapy (how are tumors rejected) that are associated with rejection may be easier to accomplish, as therapy may enhance the differences between responding and non-responding lesions and may provide useful mechanistic insights about the requirements for successful therapy. This, in turn, could aid interpretation of future studies by monitoring whether the predicted biological end-point was reached by the tumor-targeting therapy.

Therefore, we have been interested in understanding what turns an indolent immune response into a potent inflammatory reaction capable of decisively clearing the pathogenic process. The answer may extend beyond tumor immune biology. Symptomatic acute hepatitis B and C virus infection results in viral clearance while asymptomatic infections result in chronic infection [72–74]. Allograft rejection may follow an indolent course for years before acute rejection occurs [75]. Jonas Salk hypothesized half a century ago [76] that these phenomena represented facets of a similar biologic effect that he called the delayed allergy reaction. We have been wondering whether these patterns could be explained by a common immunological constant necessary for tissue destruction [35]. Evidence is mounting that independent of the triggering mechanism, downstream events leading to rejection converge into similar patterns. Global transcript analysis has provided a broad view of biological processes associated with TSD and identified convergent characteristics. Neoplastic inflammation approaches the unresolving process of chronic HCV infection [48,72,77] and it is characterized by the expression of interferon stimulated genes (ISGs). Similar signatures can be identified in liver biopsies from patients with chronic HCV infection, and in chronic allograft rejection controlled with standard immune suppression [75]. Moreover, ISGs are consistently expressed in melanoma metastases following the systemic administration of IL-2 independently of clinical outcome [18]. It therefore appears that ISGs are part of immunological processes associated with lingering unresolving inflammation. Genes associated with cytotoxic effector function are rarely expressed in chronically inflamed tissues but consistently appear when the inflammatory process causes destruction of a tumor [18,19], allograft [75], liver in HCV [77], or gut during flares of Crohn's disease [78]. By applying transcriptional profiling to serial biopsies of basal cell cancers regressing in response to treatment with the TLR7 agonist Imiquimod, we could define in a placebo-controlled double blinded randomized study the molecular components of the ICR [19] separating them from the effects of the vehicle or the biopsy itself [79]. Among them, we observed that NK cell and activated CTL function seems to predominate during the phases of acute rejection. Interestingly, comparison with other human system of immune-mediated tissue rejection suggests that this final effector pathway is common to other pathologies. Over expression of perforin, granzymes, IL-2 receptor α and β chain, IL-15 receptor, and IL-15 itself seem to be part of a general pathway that also occurs during acute rejection of renal allografts [75]. We recently summarized the common functional units associated with TSD. These include overlapping yet distinct themes that are consistently present when TSD occurs:

(i) The STAT-1/IRF-1/T-bet/IFN-γ, IL-15 path
(ii) The Granzyme A/B, TIA-1 pathway
(iii) The CXCR3 ligand chemokine pathway
(iv) The CCR5 ligand chemokine pathway

We observed their presence in different disease models. Studies in humans have identified these signatures to be associated with improved survival of patients with colon, lung, and ovarian cancer or melanoma [71,80–85]. The same patterns were observed in neoplastic lesions responsive to immunotherapy both in humans [18,19,55] and in experimental models [86]. Allografts have been studied by biopsying organs during the acute phases of rejection and several studies have reported recurrent themes [75,87–91]. In particular, Saint-Mezard *et al.* [90] analyzed three independent data set of renal biopsies identifying a robust transcriptional signature of acute allograft rejection which well summarizes most of the components of the ICR. Imanguli *et al.* [92] observed similar patterns by studying biopsies of tissues suffering chronic graft-versus-host disease and similar patterns were observed in the liver during clearance of HCV infection [93–97]. Recently, similar signatures have been observed in the destructive phases of acute cardiovascular events [98,99], chronic obstructive pulmonary disease [100], and placental villitis [101].

The study of cancer immune responsiveness using high-throughput technologies is rapidly revolutionizing the field while simultaneously contributing to understanding of the broader phenomenon of immune rejection. These developments could not have happened without direct observations performed in human tissues at relevant moments and at places were the phenomenology is specifically occurring. We contend that this approach may be applied to the study of human pathology in general, particularly in those cases when specific tissues are targeted by the disease and the biology relevant to the phenomenology is likely restricted to that area.

6.2.4 *Concepts Emerging from the Study of Degenerative Diseases of the Eye*

The eye, while a small organ, presents with a wide assortment of diseases, much of it reflective of systemic disease. Animal models are used extensively in the study of ocular disease [102,103]. It is clear that there is a need for a better understanding of human immune mechanisms. This is growing in importance as therapy for disease has become increasingly focused. This is being recognized by many who have seen great "cures" in mice but with disappointing results in man. One of the most important words today in any researcher's vocabulary is "translational" research. One aspect of this concept, simply put, is bringing the information gleaned from animal research (often not from mammals but rather from fish and even cell culture) to the clinic to be then tested on patients. The foundation upon which this concept is based, we argue, is extremely flawed. We know that pharmaceutical firms, which are so dependent on a stream of new medications and discovery of relevant pathways leading to human disease, are concerned by the recent dearth of truly novel therapeutics and by the extraordinarily few drugs "discovered" by animal work that are of use in humans. The divergence in the immune response of humans from animals is vast [104]. We have suggested that the bench-to-bedside approach is actually backwards. It would seem to make more sense to begin with studying human mechanisms and then move on to animal models. By doing so, one would be in a better position to choose animal models more relevant to the human situation. Furthermore, with the increasing recognition of differences between the immune response in mouse compared to man, approaching this from the human perspective would help the investigator decide what needs to be excluded and what can be studied [23]. Learning first from man and using discovery techniques is a very important imperative, since we often know more about mechanisms related to mouse immunology than we do the human. A recently held meeting at NIH under the auspices of the Center for Human Immunology (http://www.nhlbi.nih.gov/resources/chi) emphasized to all the attendees that we need further data to understand normal human conditions and human conditions in the diseased state [105]. This symposium emphasized many important issues. One practical issue is that while patients suffering from autoimmune disease do have many new options, pharmaceutical firms are bringing forward far fewer "first in class" drugs. It has become clear that animal models in general have been disappointing in their capacity to predict usefulness in humans. The implications of these and many other findings are that further understanding of the human situation in health and disease needs to be pursued in order to develop more effective animal models. One long-standing issue is that man and mice are separated by at least 65 million years of evolution. It is useful to evaluate the experience with human ocular inflammatory and degenerative disease and that of the animal models that exist for both.

Ocular inflammatory disease, or uveitis, is a disorder that is the cause of about 10% of severe visual handicap in the United States. It has a calculated prevalence of 112/100,000 [106], and affects mainly children as well as individuals in their economically active years. The disease can be a result of ongoing infections such as toxoplasmosis or cytomegalovirus, as is often seen in immunocompromised individuals. The inflammatory process can be anatomically classified as being in the front of the eye (anterior uveitis), the middle of the eye (intermediate uveitis), or in the back of the eye (posterior uveitis). If all areas of the eye are involved, it is then called a panuveitis. For cases of non-infectious uveitis, immunosuppression, often given systemically, is the treatment of choice.

Experimental autoimmune uveoretinitis (EAU) is an animal model uveitis. The disease is induced by immunizing animals at sites far from the globe. The antigen can be one of several antigens that can be found in the retina and retinal pigment epithelium. Based on these experiments, several markers of disease have been identified. One is the enhanced expression of IL-2 receptors on the autoaggressive cells that can be transferred to naïve hosts to induce disease. Another finding is that both TH17 and TH1 cells are capable of inducing disease, with slightly different clinical characteristics. Induction by one type of T cell as opposed to the other depends on whether microbial antigens are used as adjuvant [107]. T regs have also been evaluated in these animal models [108] and both T regs and IL-10 play a role in down-regulation of the immune response. The model has also been induced using non-T-cells methods. EAU has been used to evaluate the use of various medications to down-regulate the immune response. One of the first was the demonstration that cyclosporine was useful in down-regulating the expression of experimental uveitis [109]. Several immunosuppressive manipulations have been used, including the use of oral tolerance [110].

With such a robust experimental model for human uveitis, one might imagine that such observations have led to major advances in the diagnosis and treatment of uveitis patients. However, the differences between human and mouse immunology have restricted the translation of observations in the rodent to the human. One significant concern has been the lack of understanding of mechanisms in humans that appear to be basic to the rodent's immune system. One of the major questions still to be addressed is the observed difference between rodent and human when the IL-2 receptor is blocked. In rodents, such therapy leads to a severe autoimmune-like syndrome, leading ultimately to death. In humans, the use of daclizumab (a humanized monoclonal antibody directed against the activated moiety (Tac) of the IL-2 receptor), leads to an amelioration of sight-threatening uveitis [111]. Reliable biomarkers for uveitic activity or inflammatory control remain elusive. We have evaluated one activation marker, GITR, in uveitis patients [112]. This receptor's expression can be induced with a steroid in rodents, but not in humans. In addition, the full role of TH17 cells in human disease still needs to be better defined. We have demonstrated the presence of TH17 cells in the peripheral blood of patients with uveitis, including sarcoidosis [113]. However, the role these cells play has been put into question with the finding that TH17 cells also express T regulatory characteristics. Blocking the TH17 receptor in animals may result in the diminution of disease, but it is disconcerting that in humans a similar blockage may result into an exacerbation of disease, essentially blocking T regulatory cells. Further, the generation of TH17 cells appears to be fundamentally different in humans when compared to the rodent. While the presence of TGF-beta is needed in the rodent, this appears not to be the case for the human.

The function of T regulatory cells is an important issue that needs to be more fully explored in humans. While the FoxP3 CD4 population in mice clearly harbors a large proportion of these immunoregulatory cells, in the human we still do not have good biomarkers to definitively identify these cells. We reported that FoxP3 cells decrease in active uveitis, but these findings are extremely variable [114]. Further evidence that using the rodent model to predict biomarkers in humans is problematic can be seen with the use of Daclizumab in the treatment of uveitis, which was mentioned above.

The fact that humans are "outbred" presents very special needs in terms of the search for biomarkers. In a study of 50 uveitis patients, a pathway-specific DNA microarray was used for gene expression profiling. While several genes were differentially expressed in the uveitis patients, as compared to controls, there appeared to be at least 4 gene expression patterns. Unfortunately, these gene signatures were not found in specific disorders, but rather were associated with specific families. Further, altered gene expression was observed in the same patient during both when the disease was active and inactive. These findings emphasize the need to identify biomarkers in patients, which may be different between individuals with the same disease [115].

Recent observations have strongly supported the notion that age-related macular degeneration (AMD) is an immunologically mediated disease [116]. It is a disorder that will be reaching epidemic proportions in the next few decades [117–119]. Single nucleotide polymorphisms of CFH, as well as other parts of the complement system, have been associated with this disorder [120]. While animal models exist for AMD, it is not clear how closely they reflect the situation in humans. One model is induced using CEP immunization, and this model may provide important immune insights relevant to human disease [121]. Some data are, however, conflicting. For example, the animal models of AMD, many of which are chemokine knockouts [103], suggest that suboptimal macrophage activity leads to the disease. However, human studies would suggest that macrophage activity is actually heightened, based on the presence of TNF-alpha producing macrophages in the peripheral blood of AMD patients with choroidal neo-revascularization [122].

In summary, while animal models do provide some insight into mechanisms of human disease, it has become increasingly clear that much of the information gathered from rodent models has limited applicability to humans. A new paradigm is required; one that emphasizes the use of human studies to better define disease mechanisms. With this process of reverse engineering, a return to animal models based on human-derived knowledge would facilitate decisions about what information gleaned from animals is relevant to human disease, and what is of limited relevance. Others have gone beyond this approach of simply identifying mechanisms shared by both animal models and humans, and suggested the development and use of "humanized" animals. This approach emphasizes the study of spontaneous disease models, and uses "dirty" animals, i.e., animals that live in a normal environment rather than a clinical, germ-free laboratory environment.

6.3 Discussion and Conclusions

We hope that the two examples discussed in this chapter address the growing need for a paradigm shift in research, which is crucial if the latter is to be relevant to human disease [3,4,23]. The importance of arguments about hypothesis-driven versus discovery-driven research, or human versus animal-oriented research, fades when compared to the upstream question of how relevant the hypotheses are and the systems used to address them. Humble recognition that the goals of biomedical research do not align with rationalizations supporting projects that best fit the chance of success of individual investigators [25] is by far the most critical parameter. We should ask ourselves whether we truly believe that the problem being tackled has anything to do with human disease and suffering. With these two examples, we question hypothesis-driven research not because we believe the process is scientifically faulty, but because the hypothesis chosen is often done so superficially and is not always worth testing. We believe that observational studies should precede experimental work and no hypothesis-driven research should be funded at tax payers' expenses unless its relevance to human disease has been clearly documented from scanning human disease with inclusive genome-wide approaches. It is clear that future progress will center around understanding human mechanisms both in health and disease. The process of reverse engineering is imperative here. Biomedical research will only succeed when drug development is guided by experience gained through informative clinical trials with the purpose of not only testing the effectiveness of treatment, but also providing mechanistic insights into the differences between expected and observed results. Facts can only be gathered by a systematic approach to study design. Perhaps the consequence of this might be that fewer clinical studies will be undertaken, but those that are should give account of relevant biological questions. Perhaps less money should be spent on stabularia and other elegant animal facilities and more on studying humans to determine the questions that are then addressed in animals. Study sections should be challenged to consider the potential for human application over hypothesis-driven research, and that hypotheses are useful only when they have proven their relevance. This can only be achieved, we argue, through a courageous effort of the research community to change the way biomedical research is funded, published, and rewarded.

References

1. Horig, H., Marincola, E., and Marincola, F.M. Obstacles and opportunities in translational research. *Nat Med* 2005, 11: 705–708.
2. Littman, B.H., Di Mario, L., Plebani, M., and Marincola, F.M. What's next in translational medicine? *Clin Sci (Lond)* 2007, 112: 217–227.

3. Marincola, F.M. Translational medicine: A two way road. *J Transl Med* 2003, 1: 1.
4. Marincola, F.M. In support of descriptive studies: Relevance to translational research. *J Transl Med* 2007, 5: 21.
5. Marincola, F.M. A trouble with translational medicine. *J Intern Med* 2011, 270(2): 123–127.
6. Snyderman, R. AAP Presidential Address: The AAP and the transformation of medicine. *J Clin Invest* 2004, 114: 1169–1173.
7. Heffler, S., Smith, S., Keehan, S., Borger, C., Clemens, M.K., and Truffer, C. Trends: U.S. health spending projections For 2004–2014. *Health Aff (Millwood)* 2005.
8. Tesch, G., Amur, S., Schousboe, J.T., Siegel, J.N., Lesko, L.J., and Bai, J.P. Successes Achieved and challenges ahead in translating biomarkers into clinical applications. *AAPS J* 2010.
9. Tahara, H., Sato, M., Thurin, M., Wang, E., Butterfield, L.H., Disis, M.L., Fox, B.A., Lee, P.P., Khleif, S.N., Wigginton, J.M., *et al.* Emerging concepts in biomarker discovery; The US-Japan workshop on immunological molecular markers in oncology. *J Transl Med* 2009, 7: 45.
10. Garber, K. Cancer research. Melanoma drug vindicates targeted approach. *Science* 2009, 326: 1619.
11. Mylonakis, E., Paliou, M., and Rich, J.D. Plasma viral load testing in the management of HIV infection. *Am Fam Physician* 2001, 63: 483–486.
12. Smith, C.L. and Stein, G.E. Viral load as a surrogate end point in HIV disease. *Ann Pharmacother* 2002, 36: 280–287.
13. Roberts, L., Passmore, J.A., Williamson, C., Little, F., Bebell, L.M., Mlisana, K., Burgers, W.A., van L.F., Walzl, G., Djoba Siawaya, J.F., *et al.* Plasma cytokine levels during acute HIV-1 infection predict HIV disease progression. *AIDS* 2010.
14. Francois, C., Castelain, S., Duverlie, G., Capron, D., and Nguyen-Khac, E. Optimizing the treatment of chronic viral hepatitis C. *Expert Rev Gastroenterol Hepatol* 2009, 3: 607–613.
15. Tanaka, Y., Nishida, N., Sugiyama, M., Kurosaki, M., Matsuura, K., Sakamoto, N., Nakagawa, M., Korenaga, M., Hino, K., Hige, S., *et al.* Genome-wide association of IL28B with response to pegylated interferon-alpha and ribavirin therapy for chronic hepatitis C. *Nat Genet* 2009.
16. Thomas, D.L., Thio, C.L., Martin, M.P., Qi, Y., Ge, D., O'huigin, C., Kidd, J., Kidd, K., Khakoo, S.I., Alexander, G., *et al.* Genetic variation in IL28B and spontaneous clearance of hepatitis C virus. *Nature* 2009.

17. Lee, K.-H., Wang, E., Nielsen, M.-B., Wunderlich, J., Migueles, S., Connors, M., Steinberg, S.M., Rosenberg, S.A., and Marincola, F.M. Increased vaccine-specific T cell frequency after peptide-based vaccination correlates with increased susceptibility to *in vitro* stimulation but does not lead to tumor regression. *J Immunol* 1999, 163: 6292–6300.
18. Panelli, M.C., Wang, E., Phan, G., Puhlman, M., Miller, L., Ohnmacht, G.A., Klein, H., and Marincola, F.M. Gene-expression profiling of the response of peripheral blood mononuclear cells and melanoma metastases to systemic IL-2 administration. *Genome Biol* 2002, 3:RESEARCH0035.
19. Panelli, M.C., Stashower, M., Slade, H.B., Smith, K., Norwood, C., Abati, A., Fetsch, P.A., Filie, A., Walters, S.A., Astry, C., *et al.* Sequential gene profiling of basal cell carcinomas treated with Imiquimod in a placebo-controlled study defines the requirements for tissue rejection. *Genome Biol* 2006, 8: R8.
20. Panelli, M.C., Martin, B., Nagorsen, D., Wang, E., Smith, K., Monsurro, V., and Marincola, F.M. A genomic and proteomic-based hypothesis on the eclectic effects of systemic interleukin-2 administration in the context of melanoma-specific immunization. *Cells Tissues Organs* 2003, 177: 124–131.
21. Panelli, M.C., White, R.L. Jr, Foster, M., Martin, B., Wang, E., Smith, K., Marincola, F.M. Forecasting the cytokine storm following systemic interleukin-2 administration. *J Transl Med* 2004, 2: 17.
22. Butterfield, L.H., Disis, M.L., Fox, B.A., Lee, P.P., Khleif, S.N., Thurin, M., Trinchieri, G., Wang, E., Wigginton, J., Chaussabel, D., *et al.* A systematic approach to biomarker discovery; Preamble to 'the iSBTc-FDA taskforce on immunotherapy biomarkers'. *J Transl Med* 2008, 6: 81.
23. Nussenblatt, R.B., Marincola, F.M., and Schechter, A.N. Translational medicine—doing it backwards. *J Transl Med* 2010, 8: 12.
24. Davis, M.M. A prescription for human immunology. *Immunity* 2008, 29: 835–838.
25. Young, N.S., Ioannidis, J.P., and Al-Ubaydli, O. Why current publication practices may distort science. *PLoS Med* 2008, 5: e201.
26. Brander, C. and Marincola, F.M. AAAS joins the translational medicine family. *J Transl Med* 2009, 7: 32.
27. Rees, J. Complex disease and the new clinical sciences. *Science* 2002, 296: 698–700.
28. Lander, E.S. The new genomics: global view of biology. *Science* 1996, 274: 536–539.

29. Lander, E.S. Array of hope. *Nat Genet* 1999, 21: 3–4.
30. Cucuianu, A. Chaos in cancer? *Nat Med* 1998, 4: 1342–1343.
31. Coffey, D.S. Self-organization, complexity and chaos: The new biology for medicine. *Nat Med* 1998, 4: 882–885.
32. Callard, R., George, A.J.T., and Stark, J. Cytokines, chaos and complexity. *Cell* 1999, 11: 513.
33. Dalgleish, A. The relevance of non-linear mathematics (chaos theory) to the treatment of cancer, the role of the immune response and the potential for vaccines. *QJM* 1999, 92: 347–359.
34. Rew, D.A. Tumour biology, chaos and non-linear dynamics. *Eur J Surg Oncol* 1999, 25: 86–89.
35. Wang, E., Worschech, A., and Marincola, F.M. The immunologic constant of rejection. *Trends Immunol* 2008, 29: 256–262.
36. Wang, E., and Marincola, F.M. (Eds.) *Signatures of Rejection*. New York, NY: Springer; 2010.
37. Bialek, W. and Botstein, D. Introductory science and mathematics education for 21st-Century biologists. *Science* 2004, 303: 788–790.
38. van der Bruggen, P., Traversari, C., Chomez, P., Lurquin, C., De Plaen, E., Van den Eynde, B., Knuth, A., and Boon, T. A gene encoding an antigen recognized by cytolytic T lymphocytes on a human melanoma. *Science* 1991, 254: 1643–1647.
39. Marincola, F.M. and Ferrone, S. Immunotherapy of melanoma: The good news, the bad news and what to do next. *Sem Cancer Biol* 2003, 13: 387–389.
40. Slingluff, C.L., Jr. and Speiser, DE. Progress and controversies in developing cancer vaccines. *J Transl Med* 2005, 3: 18.
41. Monsurro', V., Wang, E., Panelli, M.C., Nagorsen, D., Jin, P., Smith, K., Ngalame, Y., Even, J., and Marincola, F.M. Active-specific immunization against melanoma: Is the problem at the receiving end? *Sem Cancer Biol* 2003, 13: 473–480.
42. Rosenberg, S.A., Yang, J.C., and Restifo, N.P. Cancer immunotherapy: moving beyond current vaccines. *Nat Med* 2004, 10: 909–915.
43. Mocellin, S., Mandruzzato, S., Bronte, V., Marincola, F.M. Correspondence 1: Cancer vaccines: Pessimism in check. *Nat Med* 2004, 10: 1278–1279.
44. Atkins, M.B., Lotze, M.T., Dutcher, J.P., Fisher, R.I., Weiss, G., Margolin, K., Abrams, J., Sznol, M., Parkinson, D.R., Hawkins, M., *et al.* High-dose recombinant interleukin-2 therapy for patients with metastatic

melanoma. Analysis of 270 patients treated between 1985 and 1993. *J Clin Oncol* 1998, 17: 2105–2116.

45. Atkins, M.B., Regan, M., and McDermott, D. Update on the role of interleukin 2 and other cytokines in the treatment of patients with stage IV renal carcinoma. *Clin Cancer Res* 2004, 10: 6342S–6346S.
46. Schwartzentruber, D.J., Lawson, D., Richards, J., Conry, R.M., Miller, D., Treisman, J., Gailani, F., Riley, L., Conlon, K., Pockaj, B.A., *et al.* A phase III multi-insitutional randomized study of immunization with the gp100:209-217(210M) peptide followed by high dose IL-2 vs high dose IL-2 alone in patients with metastatic melanoma. *N Engl J Med* 2010, submitted.
47. Marincola, F.M., Jaffe, E.M., Hicklin, D.J., and Ferrone, S. Escape of human solid tumors from T cell recognition. Molecular mechanisms and functional significance. *Adv Immunol* 2000, 74: 181–273.
48. Marincola, F.M., Wang, E., Herlyn, M., Seliger, B., and Ferrone, S. Tumors as elusive targets of T cell-based active immunotherapy. *Trends Immunol* 2003, 24: 335–342.
49. Marincola, F.M. A balanced review of the status of T cell-based therapy against cancer. *J Transl Med* 2005, 3: 16.
50. Wang, E., Selleri, S., Sabatino, M., Monaco, A., Pos, Z., Stroncek, D.F., and Marincola, F.M. Spontaneous and tumor-induced cancer rejection in humans. *Exp Opin Biol Ther* 2008, 8: 337–349.
51. Jin, P. and Wang, E. Polymorphism in clinical immunology. From HLA typing to immunogenetic profiling. *J Transl Med* 2003, 1: 8.
52. Liu, D., O'Day, S.J., Yang, D., Boasberg, P., Milford, R., Kristedja, T., Groshen, S., and Weber, J. Impact of gene polymorphisms on clinical outcome for stage IV melanoma patients treated with biochemotherapy: An exploratory study. *Clin Cancer Res* 2005, 11: 1237–1246.
53. Ugurel, S., Schrama, D., Keller, G., Schadendorf, D., Brocker, E.B., Houben, R., Zapatka, M., Fink, W., Kaufman, H.L., and Becker, J.C. Impact of the CCR5 gene polymorphism on the survival of metastatic melanoma patients receiving immunotherapy. *Cancer Immunol Immunother* 2007, 57: 685–691.
54. Sabatino, M., Kim-Schulze, S., Panelli, M.C., Stroncek, D.F., Wang, E., Tabak, B., Kim, D.-W., DeRaffele, G., Pos, Z., Marincola, F.M., *et al.* Serum vascular endothelial growth factor (VEGF) and fibronectin predict clinical response to high-dose interleukin-2 (IL-2) therapy. *J Clin Oncol* 2008, 27: 2645–2652.

55. Wang, E., Miller, L.D., Ohnmacht, G.A., Mocellin, S., Petersen, D., Zhao, Y., Simon, R., Powell, J.I., Asaki, E., Alexander, H.R., *et al.* Prospective molecular profiling of subcutaneous melanoma metastases suggests classifiers of immune responsiveness. *Cancer Res* 2002, 62: 3581–3586.
56. Wang, E., Panelli, M.C., Monsurro', V., and Marincola, F.M. Gene expression profiling of anti-cancer immune responses. *Curr Opin Mol Ther* 2004, 6: 288–295.
57. Wang, E., Panelli, M.C., and Marincola, F.M. Gene profiling of immune responses against tumors. *Curr Opin Immunol* 2005, 17: 423–427.
58. Wang, E., Panelli, M., and Marincola, F.M. Autologous tumor rejection in humans: Trimming the myths. *Immunol Invest* 2006, 35: 437–458.
59. Bittner, M., Meltzer, P., Chen, Y., Jiang, E., Seftor, E., Hendrix, M., Radmacher, M., Simon, R., Yakhini, Z., Ben-Dor, A., *et al.* Molecular classification of cutaneous malignant melanoma by gene expression: Shifting from a continuous spectrum to distinct biologic entities. *Nature* 2000, 406: 536–840.
60. Wang, E. and Marincola, F.M. A natural history of melanoma: Serial gene expression analysis. *Immunol Today* 2000, 21: 619–623.
61. Wang, E., Lichtenfels, R., Bukur, J., Ngalame, Y., Panelli, M.C., Seliger B., and Marincola, F.M. Ontogeny and oncogenesis balance the transcriptional profile of renal cell cancer. *Cancer Res* 2004, 64: 7279–7287.
62. Wang, E., Panelli, M.C., Zavaglia, K., Mandruzzato, S., Hu, N., Taylor, P.R., Seliger, B., Zanovello, P., Freedman, R.S., and Marincola, F.M. Melanoma-restricted genes. *J Transl Med* 2004, 2: 34.
63. Marincola, F.M., Hijazi, Y.M., Fetsch, P., Salgaller, M.L., Rivoltini, L., Cormier, J.N., Simonis, T.B., Duray, P.H., Herlyn, M., Kawakami, Y., *et al.* Analysis of expression of the melanoma associated antigens MART-1 and gp100 in metastatic melanoma cell lines and in *in situ* lesions. *J Immunother* 1996, 19: 192–205.
64. Cormier, J.N., Panelli, M.C., Hackett, J.A., Bettinotti, M., Mixon, A., Wunderlich, J., Parker, L., Restifo, N.P., Ferrone, S., and Marincola, F.M. Natural variation of the expression of HLA and endogenous antigen modulates CTL recognition in an *in vitro* melanoma model. *Int J Cancer* 1999, 80: 781–790.
65. Ohnmacht, G.A., Wang, E., Mocellin, S., Abati, A., Filie, A., Fetsch, P.A., Riker, A., Kammula, U.S., Rosenberg, S.A., and Marincola, F.M. Short

term kinetics of tumor antigen expression in response to vaccination. *J Immunol* 2001, 167: 1809–1820.

66. Mocellin, S., Panelli, M.C., Wang, E., Nagorsen, D., and Marincola, F.M. The dual role of IL-10. *Trends Immunol* 2002, 24: 36–43.
67. Taniguchi, T. Transcription factors IRF-1 and IRF-2: linking the immune responses and tumor suppression. *J Cell Physiol* 1997, 173: 128–130.
68. Monsurro', V., Beghelli, S., Wang, R., Barbi, S., Coin, S., Di Pasquale, G., Bersani, S., Castellucci, M., Sorio, C., Eleuteri, S., *et al.* Anti-viral status segregates two pancreatic adenocarcinoma molecular phenotypes with potential relevance for adenoviral gene therapy. *J Transl Med* 2009, in press.
69. Wallace, T.A., Prueitt, R.L., Yi, M., Howe, T.M., Gillespie, J.W., Yfantis, H.G., Stephens, R.M., Caporaso, N.E., Loffredo, C.A., Ambs, S. Tumor immunobiological differences in prostate cancer between African-American and European-American men. *Cancer Res* 2008, 68: 927–936.
70. Martin, D.N., Boersma, B.J., Yi, M., Reimers, M., Howe, T.M., Yfantis, H.G., Tsai, Y.C., Williams, E.H., Lee, D.H., Stephens, R.M., *et al.* Differences in the tumor microenvironment between African-American and European-American breast cancer patients. *PLoS ONE* 2009, 4: e4531.
71. Galon, J., Costes, A., Sanchez-Cabo, F., Kirilovsky, A., Mlecnik, B., Lagorce-Pages, C., Tosolini, M., Camus, M., Berger, A., Wind, P., *et al.* Type, density, and location of immune cells within human colorectal tumors predict clinical outcome. *Science* 2006, 313: 1960–1964.
72. Bowen, D.G. and Walker, C.M. Adaptive immune responses in acute and chronic hepatitis C virus infection. *Nature* 2005, 436: 946–952.
73. Hardin, J.A. Dendritic cells: Potential triggers of autoimmunity and targets for therapy. *Ann Rheum Dis* 2005, 64 Suppl 4: iv86–iv90.
74. Rehermann, B. and Nascimbeni, M. Immunology of hepatitis B virus and hepatitis C virus infection. *Nat Rev Immunol* 2005, 5: 215–229.
75. Sarwal, M., Chua, M.S., Kambham, N., Hsieh, S.C., Satterwhite, T., Masek, M., and Salvatierra, O., Jr. Molecular heterogeneity in acute renal allograft rejection identified by DNA microarray profiling. *N Engl J Med* 2003, 349: 125–138.
76. Salk, J. Immunological paradoxes: Theoretical considerations in the rejection or retention of grafts, tumors, and normal tissue. *Ann N Y Acad Sci* 1969, 164: 365–380.
77. Smith, M.W., Yue, Z.N., Korth, M.J., Do, H.A., Boix, L., Fausto, N., Bruix, J., Carithers, R.L., Jr., and Katze, M.G. Hepatitis C virus and liver disease:

Global transcriptional profiling and identification of potential markers. *Hepatology* 2003, 38: 1458–1467.

78. Netea, M.G., Azam, T., Ferwerda, G., Girardin, S.E., Walsh, M., Park, J.S., Abraham, E., Kim, J.M., Yoon, D.Y., Dinarello, C.A., *et al.* IL-32 synergizes with nucleotide oligomerization domain (NOD) 1 and NOD2 ligands for IL-1beta and IL-6 production through a caspase 1-dependent mechanism. *Proc Natl Acad Sci USA* 2005, 102:16309–16314.
79. Deonarine, K., Panelli, M.C., Stashower, M.E., Jin, P., Smith, K., Slade, H.B., Norwood, C., Wang, E., Marincola, F.M., and Stroncek, D.F. Gene expression profiling of cutaneous wound healing. *J Transl Med* 2007, 5: 11.
80. Benencia, F., Courreges, M.C., Conejo-Garcia, J.R., Mohamed-Hadley, A., Zhang, L., Buckanovich, R.J., Carroll, R., Fraser, N., and Coukos, G. HSV oncolytic therapy upregulates interferon-inducible chemokines and recruits immune effector cells in ovarian cancer. *Mol Ther* 2005, 12: 789–802.
81. Pages, F., Berger, A., Camus, M., Sanchez-Cabo, F., Costes, A., Molidor, R., Mlecnik, B., Kirilovsky, A., Nilsson, M., Damotte, D., *et al.* Effector memory T cells, early metastasis, and survival in colorectal cancer. *N Engl J Med* 2005, 353: 2654–2666.
82. Dieu-Nosjean, M.C., Antoine, M., Danel, C., Heudes, D., Wislez, M., Poulot, V., Rabbe, N., Laurans, L., Tartour, E., de, C.L., *et al.* Long-term survival for patients with non-small-cell lung cancer with intratumoral lymphoid structures. *J Clin Oncol* 2008, 26: 4410–4417.
83. Camus, M., Tosolini, M., Mlecnik, B., Pages, F., Kirilovsky, A., Berger, A., Costes, A., Bindea, G., Charoentong, P., Bruneval, P., *et al.* Coordination of intratumoral immune reaction and human colorectal cancer recurrence. *Cancer Res* 2009, 69: 2685–2693.
84. Galon, J., Fridman, W.H., and Pages, F. The adaptive immunologic microenvironment in colorectal cancer: A novel perspective. *Cancer Res* 2007, 67: 1883–1886.
85. Harlin, H., Meng, Y., Peterson, A.C., Zha, Y., Tretiakova, M., Slingluff, C., McKee, M., and Gajewski, T.F. Chemokine expression in melanoma metastases associated with CD8+ T-cell recruitment. *Cancer Res* 2009, 69: 3077–3085.
86. Shanker, A., Verdeil, G., Buferne, M., Inderberg-Suso, E.M., Puthier, D., Joly, F., Nguyen, C., Leserman, L., uphan-Anezin, N., Schmitt-Verhulst, A.M. CD8 T cell help for innate antitumor immunity. *J Immunol* 2007, 179: 6651–6662.

87. Hardstedt, M., Finnegan, C.P., Kirchhof, N., Hyland, K.A., Wijkstrom, M., Murtaugh, M.P., Hering, B.J. Post-transplant upregulation of chemokine messenger RNA in non-human primate recipients of intraportal pig islet xenografts. *Xenotransplantation* 2005, 12: 293–302.

88. Karason, K., Jernas, M., Hagg, D.A., and Svensson, P.A. Evaluation of CXCL9 and CXCL10 as circulating biomarkers of human cardiac allograft rejection. *BMC Cardiovasc Disord* 2006, 6: 29.

89. Reeve, J., Einecke, G., Mengel, M., Sis, B., Kayser, N., Kaplan, B., Halloran, P.F. Diagnosing rejection in renal transplants: A comparison of molecular- and histopathology-based approaches. *Am J Transplant* 2009, 9: 1802–1810.

90. Saint-Mezard, P., Berthier, C.C., Zhang, H., Hertig, A., Kaiser, S., Schumacher, M., Wieczorek, G., Bigaud, M., Kehren, J., Rondeau, E., *et al.* Analysis of independent microarray datasets of renal biopsies identifies a robust transcript signature of acute allograft rejection. *Transpl Int* 2009, 22: 293–302.

91. Hama, N., Yanagisawa, Y., Dono, K., Kobayashi, S., Marubashi, S., Nagano, H., Umeshita, K., Watanabe, S., Uchiyama, Y., and Monden, M. Gene expression profiling of acute cellular rejection in rat liver transplantation using DNA microarrays. *Liver Transpl* 2009, 15: 509–521.

92. Imanguli, M.M., Swaim, W.D., League, S.C., Gress, R.E., Pavletic, S.Z., and Hakim, F.T. Increased T-bet+ cytotoxic effectors and type I interferon-mediated processes in chronic graft-versus-host disease of the oral mucosa. *Blood* 2009, 113: 3620–3630.

93. Bigger, C.B., Brasky, K.M., and Lanford, R.E. DNA microarray analysis of chimpanzee liver during acute resolving hepatitis C virus infection. *J Virol* 2001, 75: 7059–7066.

94. He, X.S., Ji, X., Hale, M.B., Cheung, R., Ahmed, A., Guo, Y., Nolan, G.P., Pfeffer, L.M., Wright, T.L., Risch, N., *et al.* Global transcriptional response to interferon is a determinant of HCV treatment outcome and is modified by race. *Hepatology* 2006, 44: 352–359.

95. Feld, J.J., Nanda, S., Huang, Y., Chen, W., Cam, M., Pusek, S.N., Schweigler, L.M., Theodore, D., Zacks, S.L., Liang, T.J., *et al.* Hepatic gene expression during treatment with peginterferon and ribavirin: Identifying molecular pathways for treatment response. *Hepatology* 2007, 46: 1548–1563.

96. Nanda, S., Havert, M.B., Calderon, G.M., Thomson, M., Jacobson, C., Kastner, D., and Liang, T.J. Hepatic transcriptome analysis of hepatitis

C virus infection in chimpanzees defines unique gene expression patterns associated with viral clearance. *PLoS ONE* 2008, 3: e3442.

97. Asselah, T., Bieche, I., Narguet, S., Sabbagh, A., Laurendeau, I., Ripault, M.P., Boyer, N., Martinot-Peignoux, M., Valla, D., Vidaud, M., *et al.* Liver gene expression signature to predict response to pegylated interferon plus ribavirin combination therapy in patients with chronic hepatitis C. *Gut* 2008, 57: 516–524.
98. Zhao, D.X., Hu, Y., Miller, G.G., Luster, A.D., Mitchell, R.N., and Libby, P. Differential expression of the IFN-gamma-inducible CXCR3-binding chemokines, IFN-inducible protein 10, monokine induced by IFN, and IFN-inducible T cell alpha chemoattractant in human cardiac allografts: Association with cardiac allograft vasculopathy and acute rejection. *J Immunol* 2002, 169: 1556–1560.
99. Okamoto, Y., Folco, E.J., Minami, M., Wara, A.K., Feinberg, M.W., Sukhova, G.K., Colvin, R.A., Kihara, S., Funahashi, T., Luster, A.D., *et al.* Adiponectin inhibits the production of CXC receptor 3 chemokine ligands in macrophages and reduces T-lymphocyte recruitment in atherogenesis. *Circ Res* 2008, 102: 218–225.
100. Costa, C., Rufino, R., Traves, S.L., Lapa, E., Silva, J.R., Barnes, P.J., and Donnelly, L.E. CXCR3 and CCR5 chemokines in induced sputum from patients with COPD. *Chest* 2008, 133: 26–33.
101. Kim, M.J., Romero, R., Kim, C.J., Tarca, A.L., Chhauy, S., LaJeunesse, C., Lee, D.C., Draghici, S., Gotsch, F., Kusanovic, J.P., *et al.* Villitis of unknown etiology is associated with a distinct pattern of chemokine up-regulation in the feto-maternal and placental compartments: Implications for conjoint maternal allograft rejection and maternal anti-fetal graft-versus-host disease. *J Immunol* 2009, 182: 3919–3927.
102. Caspi, R.R. Experimental autoimmune uveoretinitis in the rat and mouse. *Curr Protoc Immunol* 2003, Chapter 15: Unit.
103. Ding, X., Patel, M., and Chan, C.C. Molecular pathology of age-related macular degeneration. *Prog Retin Eye Res* 2009, 28: 1–18.
104. Mestas, J. and Hughes, C.C. Of mice and not men: Differences between mouse and human immunology. *J Immunol* 2004, 172: 2731–2738.
105. Nussenblatt, R.B., Bielekova, B., Childs, R., Krensky, A., Strober, W., and Trinchieri, G. National Institutes of Health Center for Human Immunology Conference, September 2009. *Ann N Y Acad Sci* 2010, 1200 Suppl 1: E1–E23.

106. Gritz, D.C. and Wong, I.G. Incidence and prevalence of uveitis in northern California: the Northern California Epidemiology of Uveitis Study. *Ophthalmology* 2004, 111: 491–500.

107. Hirota, K., Martin, B., and Veldhoen, M. Development, regulation and functional capacities of Th17 cells. *Semin Immunopathol* 2010, 32: 3–16.

108. Luger, D., Silver, P.B., Tang, J., Cua, D., Chen, Z., Iwakura, Y., Bowman, E.P., Sgambellone, N.M., Chan, C.C., and Caspi, R.R. Either a Th17 or a Th1 effector response can drive autoimmunity: Conditions of disease induction affect dominant effector category. *J Exp Med* 2008, 205: 799–810.

109. Nussenblatt, R.B. and Palestine, A.G. Cyclosporine: Immunology, pharmacology and therapeutic uses. *Surv Ophthalmol* 1986, 31: 159–169.

110. Dana, R., Nussenblatt, R., and Gordon, L. Advances in immunology: From bench to bedside—a symposium at the 2005 Annual Meeting of the Federation of Clinical Immunology Societies(FOCIS), Boston, MA, USA. *Ocul Immunol Inflamm* 2006, 14: 1–6.

111. Nussenblatt, R.B., Fortin, E., Schiffman, R., Rizzo, L., Smith, J., Van, V.P., Sran, P., Yaffe, A., Goldman, C.K., Waldmann, T.A., *et al.* Treatment of noninfectious intermediate and posterior uveitis with the humanized anti-Tac mAb: A phase I/II clinical trial. *Proc Natl Acad Sci USA* 1999, 96: 7462–7466.

112. Li, Z., Mahesh, S.P., Kim, B.J., Buggage, R.R., and Nussenblatt, R.B. Expression of glucocorticoid induced TNF receptor family related protein (GITR) on peripheral T cells from normal human donors and patients with non-infectious uveitis. *J Autoimmun* 2003, 21: 83–92.

113. madi-Obi, A., Yu, C.R., Liu, X., Mahdi, R.M., Clarke, G.L., Nussenblatt, R.B., Gery, I., Lee, Y.S., and Egwuagu, C.E. TH17 cells contribute to uveitis and scleritis and are expanded by IL-2 and inhibited by IL-27/STAT1. *Nat Med* 2007, 13: 711–718.

114. Yeh, S., Li, Z., Forooghian, F., Hwang, F.S., Cunningham, M.A., Pantanelli, S., Lew, J.C., Wroblewski, K.K., Vitale, S., and Nussenblatt, R.B. CD4+Foxp3+ T-regulatory cells in noninfectious uveitis. *Arch Ophthalmol* 2009, 127: 407–413.

115. Li, Z., Liu, B., Maminishkis, A., Mahesh, S.P., Yeh, S., Lew, J., Lim, W.K., Sen, H.N., Clarke, G., Buggage, R., *et al.* Gene expression profiling in autoimmune noninfectious uveitis disease. *J Immunol* 2008, 181: 5147–5157.

116. Nussenblatt, R.B. and Ferris, F. Age-related macular degeneration and the immune response: implications for therapy. *Am J Ophthalmol* 2007, 144: 618–626.

117. Cook, H.L., Patel, P.J., and Tufail, A. Age-related macular degeneration: Diagnosis and management. *Br Med Bull* 2008, 85: 127–149.

118. Friedman, D.S., O'Colmain, B.J., Munoz, B., Tomany, S.C., McCarty, C., de Jong, P.T., Nemesure, B., Mitchell, P., and Kempen, J. Prevalence of age-related macular degeneration in the United States. *Arch Ophthalmol* 2004, 122: 564–572.

119. Klein, R., Peto, T., Bird, A., and Vannewkirk, M.R. The epidemiology of age-related macular degeneration. *Am J Ophthalmol* 2004, 137: 486–495.

120. Hageman, G.S., Anderson, D.H., Johnson, L.V., Hancox, L.S., Taiber, A.J., Hardisty, L.I., Hageman, J.L., Stockman, H.A., Borchardt, J.D., Gehrs, K.M., *et al.* A common haplotype in the complement regulatory gene factor H (HF1/CFH) predisposes individuals to age-related macular degeneration. *Proc Natl Acad Sci USA* 2005, 102: 7227–7232.

121. Hollyfield, J.G., Bonilha, V.L., Rayborn, M.E., Yang, X., Shadrach, K.G., Lu, L., Ufret, R.L., Salomon, R.G., and Perez, V.L. Oxidative damage-induced inflammation initiates age-related macular degeneration. *Nat Med* 2008, 14: 194–198.

122. Cousins, S.W., Espinosa-Heidmann, D.G., and Csaky, K.G. Monocyte activation in patients with age-related macular degeneration. A biomarker of risk for choroidal neovascularization? *Arch Ophthalmol* 2004, 122: 1013–1018.

Chapter 7

Imaging Biomarkers for Innovative Drug Development: Translation from Bench to Bedside and Back

Jingsong Wang
Head of China R&D and Head of Translational Medicine Asia Pacific at Sanofi
31F, Tower 1, Plaza 66, 1266 Nanjing Road West, Shanghai 200040, China
jingsong.wang@sanofi.com

7.1 Introduction

Imaging biomarkers are measurable characteristics obtained through imaging technologies that indicate a specific biological process is occurring in the body. Compared with biochemical, molecular, and histological biomarkers, imaging biomarkers have the advantage of being non-invasive as well as spatially and temporally resolved. They provide a unique form of information to compliment traditional techniques and measurements, including a drug's pharmacokinetics and distribution profile and interaction with its target. Imaging biomarkers have the capability to provide a direct pathophysiological correlation between disease mechanism and therapy. The read-outs obtained using imaging biomarkers

Translational Medicine: The Future of Therapy
Edited by James Mittra and Christopher-Paul Milne

ISBN 978-981-4316-99-6 (Hardback), 978-981-4364-84-3 (eBook)
www.panstanford.com

are therefore potentially the closest analogs to clinical outcomes. They help speed the process of drug development as the functional imaging shows effectiveness earlier than any anatomic changes. Additionally, the role of imaging in patient diagnostics and management is well established. It is quite fitting that imaging biomarkers play an increasing role in both drug development and patient care in multiple disease areas.

Although remarkable progress has been made in introducing cutting edge technologies in imaging biomarker development to the bench, significant challenges remain in translating this knowledge into the clinical drug development at the bedside. In this chapter, I illustrate the current state-of-the-art and emerging challenges for research work at the bench, clinical translation, and eventual application of imaging biomarkers for the development of innovative therapeutics to treat human diseases.

7.2 The Different Types of Imaging Biomarkers

There are two major types of imaging platforms: anatomical and functional imaging. Anatomical imaging identifies anatomic structures in the body and mainly includes conventional radiography (X-ray), ultrasonography (ultrasound), computer tomography (CT), and magnetic resonance imaging (MRI). Molecular imaging, in contrast, visualizes, characterizes, and quantifies not just anatomical structures but also physiological processes at the cellular and subcellular levels with exquisite spatial, temporal, and biochemical resolution *in situ* and *in vivo* with radiolabeled probes or radiotracers that interact with protein targets within or on the surface of the cells [1]. It utilizes a variety of technologies, such as positron emission tomography (PET), single photo-emission computed tomography (SPECT), CT, MRI, ultrasound, optical, and associated imaging agents.

PET imaging, which uses tracers labeled with positron-emitting radioisotopes such as ^{18}F-fluorodeoxyglucose (FDG), is the most common used molecular imaging approach in the clinical realm. PET-based molecular imaging technique is a powerful methodology that facilitates understanding of the molecular basis of disease and optimal characterization of the biological process at the cellular level that underlies pathological states. The introduction of FDG to detect and measure regional glucose metabolism (as a biomarker for function) by investigators at The University of Pennsylvania in 1976 opened the door to utilizing this powerful technique in clinical practice and drug development for multiple therapeutic areas. In select diseases, it has already been used to measure efficacy early in treatment. In particular, the impact of FDG-PET in oncology has been extraordinary [2]. Furthermore, PET imaging requires a minimal amount of drug (<1 nmol) because of the strong association between the PET signal and concentration of the radiolabeled drug. This makes it feasible to carry out microdosing studies to evaluate pharmacokinetics and pharmacodynamics at the initial stage of clinical development.

In the preclinical setting, varieties of imaging modalities are actively being developed as biomarkers. For example, recent data show that contrast-enhanced ultrasound imaging with molecularly targeted microbubbles can be used to monitor angiogenic marker expression during tumor growth [3]. The ultrasound microbubbles targeted with one of several antibodies — anti-integrin, anti-endoglin, or anti-vascular endothelial growth factor receptor 2 — were injected into mice with implanted breast, ovarian, or pancreatic tumors. Changes in the relative uptake of each targeted microbubble reflected changes in the angiogenic mechanisms of the tumor at different stages of its growth. This opens the possibility of *in vivo* molecular profiling of tumor angiogenesis not just as a diagnostic tool but also as a foundation for providing personalized treatment for cancer patients [4]. This is especially important in light of the expanding menu of anti-angiogenesis therapies. Current imaging techniques for angiogenesis, such as dynamic CT, MRI, and conventional color or power Doppler, are nonspecific with regard to molecular angiogenic pathways. Molecular targeted ultrasound has the potential to help select what agents should be administered to whom and in what order.

With more novel molecular targets being identified for various diseases, the availability of sophisticated and multifunctional contrast agents and advances in the development of new technologies and instrumentations have led to multi-modality molecular imaging platforms becoming the area of focus for preclinical imaging biomarker development. Contrast-enhanced molecular ultrasound with molecularly targeted contrast microbubbles is being explored as a clinically translatable molecular imaging strategy. Optical imaging with fluorescent molecular probes, and ultrasound imaging with molecularly targeted microbubbles, are attractive approaches as they provide real-time imaging, are relatively inexpensive, produce images with high spatial resolution, and do not involve ionizing irradiation. Raman spectroscopy/microscopy has emerged as a molecular optical imaging strategy for ultrasensitive detection of multiple chemical compounds or biomolecules with both *in vivo* and *ex vivo* versatility. Photoacoustic imaging is a hybrid of optical and ultrasound techniques that utilizes optically excitable molecularly targeted contrast agents and quantitative detection of resulting oscillatory contrast agent movement using ultrasound. These activities, coupled with advances in instrumentation such as endoscopes and microcatheters, will propel these techniques to the forefront of the preclinical development and clinical translation of imaging biomarkers [5].

7.2.1 *Drug Development and Imaging Biomarkers*

Quantitative imaging techniques allow for the use of imaging biomarkers to increase the efficiency, effectiveness, and speed of the drug development process by providing early identification of promising candidate drugs. Imaging biomarkers can be used in a variety of ways in the drug development process, such as target validation, confirmation of mechanism of action, pharmacokinetics assessment to support optimal dose selection, patient stratification in clinical trials, and early measure of clinical activity. They are generally used as a valuable tool to guide go/no go decision making in the drug development process. However, in certain situations they can also be used as surrogate markers to assess efficacy in the context of regulatory filing.

Surrogate markers are a subset of biomarkers that have been shown to accurately predict clinical efficacy. Surrogate biomarker status marks the ultimate success for clinical translation, and represents the Holy Grail of biomarker development. In order to qualify as a surrogate biomarker, imaging biomarkers must be standardized and qualified in well-controlled clinical studies and multicenter settings and be shown to be reliably correlated with the disease activity. Surrogate imaging endpoints are particularly useful when relevant clinical outcomes are not measurable in the time frame of the clinical trial.

Imaging biomarkers play a particularly important role in the drug development for chronic complex diseases such as Alzheimer's disease (AD), chronic obstructive pulmonary disease (COPD), and osteoarthritis (OA), since longer treatment duration is needed to observe any therapeutic effect in clinical trials for these diseases [6].

7.2.2 *Imaging Biomarkers in Preclinical Studies*

Preclinical testing forms the necessary platform to investigate cutting edge imaging techniques, and serves as the launching pad for imaging biomarker development. Imaging platforms in the preclinical setting allows investigators to obtain much more information from each animal and enables noninvasive collection of data at serial time points on the same animal. This leads to a significant improvement in animal welfare as well as a reduction in the overall number of animals used. More traditional imaging modalities, such as CT and MRI, have routinely been used in animal studies. However, newer imaging modalities, especially *in vivo* molecular imaging ranging from optical MR to PET scanning, provides insights into target validation and disease mechanism dissection that are critical in preclinical studies at the bench.

Utilization of imaging biomarkers in preclinical animal models is likely to add further validity and confidence to their clinical translation. Furthermore, the ability to develop quantitative assays of pathological markers on small animals allows researchers to generate the first proof of biological activity of a specific drug candidate and also validate such information using post mortem histology. Thus, imaging biomarkers are an important tool for translational research that bridge preclinical research to clinical development [7].

However, the value of the imaging data generated pre-clinically has been limited by inadequate clinical translatability of animal models and lack of full understanding of human pathophysiology. Despite this limitation, the imaging biomarker is uniquely positioned at the preclinical stage to facilitate better translation from animal models to human subjects in clinical studies, and thereby enhance the translational research process [8]. In this regard, preclinical studies provide an outstanding opportunity to dissect the connectivity between imaging biomarkers and molecular pathways, and in turn help to better understand the pathogenesis of human diseases. This knowledge will eventually contribute to the development of better imaging modalities for use in the clinic.

7.2.3 *Clinical Translation of Imaging Biomarkers in Drug Development*

The general set-up and operation model for utilizing imaging biomarkers in drug research & development varies between pharmaceutical companies. However, the overarching strategy appears to be somewhat aligned. The common challenges faced by the drug developers are, which imaging modality is the most suitable, and when is the optimal time to incorporate imaging biomarkers into the drug development program?

The assessment for the utility of imaging biomarkers starts with evaluating the mechanism of action for the drug candidate and the potential target disease. The need for imaging biomarkers has to be carefully evaluated to ensure differentiated value is added over other forms of biomarkers. In this context, imaging biomarkers could provide the ability to avoid invasive procedures, or to report a signal earlier than other markers or clinical end points, or to serve as an initial screen that can be followed up with a more definitive molecular and/or pathological validation [7]. Whenever possible, molecular assays that can serve as surrogates for specific imaging platforms should be investigated initially. For example, the GLUT-1 test can be used as a feasibility test for FDG-PET, or a thymidine-kinase assay for FLT-PET. Preclinical imaging will be evaluated as the lead compound is being nominated. Activities to utilize imaging biomarkers in preclinical animal models will then be carried out. The clinical translation of the preclinical imaging work usually starts before the drug candidate advances to the clinical development stage.

When assessing the potential for clinical application of the imaging biomarkers, their capability to fulfill specific needs of the drug development program and clinical translatability of the imaging techniques are the most important factors to consider. For instance, while X-ray, MRI, and ultrasound imaging modalities are widely used in the clinic, human applications of optical imaging are severely hampered by the scattering and absorption of photons, which restricts applications only to the study of superficial structures [9].

Special attention needs to be paid if molecular imaging is being considered. The development of molecular imaging requires the careful coordination and integration of many disciplines, including biology, chemistry, pharmacology, medical imaging physics, applied computer sciences, and mathematics, as well as bioinformatics. The process of developing a specific tracer is complex, and resembles that for drug discovery. It is important to begin the tracer discovery effort early at the drug candidate lead identification stage, and then continue optimization of the tracer in parallel with the drug candidate. PET tracers need to be clinically validated prior to Phase I clinical trials so that they can be incorporated into early clinical development programs [1].

The type of imaging biomarker selected will impact on the clinical trial design and execution, particularly the study budget, inclusion and exclusion criteria, data analysis, site selection, and timeline. In general, imaging biomarkers will start to be used in clinical studies (most likely Phase Ib and II) with a diseased patient population in which the disease state or loci and pharmacodynamics can be monitored. An exception might be made when a microdosing study is being considered. In this context, a radiolabeled compound may be used in healthy subjects to generate pharmacokinetics and biodistribution information with PET imaging. To ensure the successful application of the imaging biomarker to the clinical trial, standardization of imaging acquisition protocols and harmonization of image analysis procedure will be part of the overall feasibility assessment. This aspect of the work is usually done through collaboration with leading clinical research centers, experienced imaging sites, and central reading facilities.

In comparison to most clinical end points, imaging biomarkers in many cases are more expensive, require complex data analysis schemes, and lack clinical validation. In general, imaging biomarker data are initially used for the evaluation of proof of mechanism and for internal decision making. Only the data on regulatory approved surrogate imaging biomarkers can be used for initial drug registration. In cases where clinical efficacy end points are easy to monitor and require a shorter treatment duration, imaging biomarkers will not be used as a primary outcome for drug registration. In this context, data on imaging biomarker will only be used for additional indications when the initial marketing approval has been obtained. The regulatory approval process for disease-modifying antirheumatic drugs (DMARDs) for RA would follow such path. Initial approval for DMARDs is based on clinical efficacy outcome, which consists of a composite score on objective and subjective disease activities [American College of Rheumatology (ACR) 20, 50 and 70], and an additional indication for preventing structural damage can be obtained with data on imaging biomarkers (e.g., using X-ray) from patient cohorts treated for at least 1 year [10].

At present, pharmaceutical companies are more likely to have internal imaging biomarker experts to oversee or coordinate the application of imaging biomarkers in drug development programs. Many companies have an internal preclinical imaging group to carry out work on animal models with discovery teams for projects at the early stage. Clinical translation assessment and the clinical integration strategy will likely be guided by a group of experts, both internal and external, in the areas of imaging technology and clinical development. At this stage, external vendors will be used for imaging data collection and analysis and other aspects of the clinical trial operation.

7.3 Experience of Imaging Biomarker Clinical Translation for Select Diseases

Significant experiences have been gained in translating and applying imaging biomarkers in clinical drug development. The following sections briefly describe the general status of imaging biomarker development in select disease areas to illustrate the success achieved, challenges ahead, and lessons that can be learned.

7.3.1 *Oncology*

With increasing understanding of cancer-related pathways and emerging discoveries of targeted signal transduction inhibitors for cancer treatment, novel pharmacodynamic endpoints of treatment efficacy are required [11]. At present, CT and MRI are the imaging biomarker technologies of choice to assess clinical changes in tumor size. While they provide superb anatomic resolution, physiological changes in the tumor microenvironment need to be assessed by dynamic contrast enhanced MRI (DCEMRI), while metabolic endpoints need to be established with PET and other molecular imaging modalities [12].

In the clinical trial setting, CT or MRI measurements of changes in tumor volume are based on the "Response Evaluation Criteria in Solid Tumours" (RECIST) criteria. These anatomical biomarkers are the only imaging surrogate endpoints that are accepted for drug product registration. However, these anatomical biomarkers are suboptimal for assessing the effect of targeted treatments that do not cause regression of tumor volume, but rather increase the extent of tumor necrosis. A number of biomarkers obtained with other imaging modalities, including PET, contrast-enhanced CT, perfusion CT and MRI, diffusion-weighted MRI, MR elastography, and spectroscopy, have the potential to establish novel parameters to complement or even replace the RECIST criteria [13].

Novel techniques for improved spatial resolution, automated quantitative methods for anatomic assessment, and development of physiological, metabolic, and molecular imaging probes are currently under active investigation [14]. Among them, PET- and SPECT-based platforms have generated the most significant impact on oncology drug development. As part of the continued maturation of the techniques and platforms, there are four key biological mechanisms that PET tracers are being developed to target: angiogenesis, hypoxia, cell proliferation, and apoptosis. However, these aforementioned techniques are not necessarily straightforward.

For example, in the case of diffusion-weighted MRI in the liver, respiratory motion can make it difficult to track the tiny movements of water molecules, requiring breath-holds in the patient. Eating has also been shown to influence diffusion MRI results, and certain apparent diffusion coefficient (ADC) measurements may be sensitive to perfusion. Therefore, important efforts of qualification and standardization remain to be done before the acceptance of some of these functional biomarkers as surrogate endpoints.

7.3.2 *Neurological and Psychological Diseases*

Molecular imaging modalities have become powerful tools for drug discovery and development in the neuroscience area due to the inaccessibility of the brain and the lack of central nervous system (CNS) specific markers to drive specific dosing. PET and SPECT scanning have the capability to directly measure alterations in regional metabolism, blood flow, or dopamine function. They are actively being employed to determine the optimal clinical dose and the pharmacokinetic profile of psychotropics by investigating the index of drug occupancy at its action sites [15]. The availability of PET ligands for essentially every neurotransmitter system constitutes a rich basis for the application of molecular imaging biomarkers in drug development for diseases of the CNS, especially AD [16]. The most recent development in the area has been the utilization of PET imaging with ^{11}C-Pittsburg compound B (PIB), a PET tracer binding to fibrillar amyloid-β deposits in the brain, to monitor the pharmacodynamic effects of bapineuzumab [17].

For Parkinson's disease, PET and SPECT can help confirm the diagnosis of parkinsonian disorders, where this is in doubt, and provide potential biomarkers for tracing the effects of putative neuroprotective and restorative agents on disease progression. PET can also confirm whether novel therapeutics have reached their intended targets and generate dose-occupancy profiles. Finally, PET and SPECT can indirectly monitor changes in brain dopamine levels and subsequently shed light on the pharmacology underlying treatment-associated complications.

More broadly, molecular imaging biomarkers can play multiple roles in drug development for dementia: (1) as a cognitive neuroscience research tool; (2) for prediction of which normal or slightly impaired individuals will develop dementia and over what time frame; (3) for early diagnosis of AD in demented individuals (sensitivity), and differentiation of AD from other form of dementia (specificity); (4) for monitoring of disease progression; and (5) for monitoring response to therapies [18]. However, no single imaging modality is yet ideal, as all involve trade-offs of speed, cost, and accuracy. Functional imaging is best suited to monitor symptomatic therapy response, and anatomic imaging or amyloid PET are more suited for use in dementia modulation studies. However, at the present time, no single measure has sufficient proven reliability, replicability, or robustness to replace clinical primary outcome end points.

At present, the broader application of molecular imaging biomarkers has been limited by the availability of radiotracers as well as comparatively low resolution. Functional MRI (fMRI) in a way overcomes these problems, but the measures obtained (the BOLD signal) are only indirect reflections of neuronal activity. Furthermore (and given the presence of cognitive problems in many patients with PD), patients need to be able to participate in tasks whilst in the scanner. Resting state fMRI is an emerging technique that does not require specific task performance and has been used to evaluate basal ganglia circuitry [19]. To date, its significance in PD or other neurodegenerative disorders has not been established.

7.3.3 *Asthma*

Clinical symptoms and lung function test (LFT) spirometry are the main conventional end points used for developing therapeutics to treat asthma. However, CT and high resolution CT (HRCT) have been introduced with different breathing maneuvers to assess the presence and severity of air trapping. Gaseous MRI contrast agents have also become available to provide a new technique for visualizing lung ventilation without ionizing radiation exposure [20]. Samee and his colleagues have shown that MRI of lungs in patients with asthma who have inhaled hyperpolarized helium-3 (HHe3) reveals ventilation defects that are well correlated with lung function and worsen with the introduction of either methacholine or exercise [21]. This sequential imaging of the lungs provides a valuable tool to investigate how the obstruction develops, and has the potential to be a powerful biomarker to characterize the subtypes of the disease and to monitor the effect of treatment. Currently, the clinical application of hyperpolarized helium MRI is limited by economics, logistics, and regulatory constraints, and is only available in a small number of medical centers. More work is needed to be done before it can be routinely used in drug development.

7.3.4 *Chronic Obstructive Pulmonary Disease*

Current regulatory-approved clinical end points assessed by spirometry measure only the general disease activity but fail to reflect the structural changes that occur at parenchyma and airway walls. This information is critically important to monitor the efficacy of disease modifying drugs for COPD. Traditional radiography has multiple limitations in measuring emphysema, which includes low specificity and sensitivity in mild cases, considerable interobserver variability, and inability to quantify the outcome. On the other hand, CT, especially HRCT, is superior to chest radiography in demonstrating the presence, distribution, and extent of emphysema [22].

Work is currently ongoing to assess the potential role of CT scanning images as a biomarker for severity of airway wall inflammation and airway obstruction in patients with COPD. At this point, the application of quantitative CT scanning to clinical studies has been used predominantly to assess the outcome of lung-volume reduction surgery, and utilization of the techniques to pharmaceutical clinical trials has obtained less conclusive results [23].

Patient populations with early, mild emphysema are the likely target for the development of disease modifying drugs. It is important to note that in comparison to functional assessment of emphysema measured by spirometry, sensitivity of HRCT to detecting early emphysematous changes is low but its accuracy is high [24]. However, the ability to assess mild emphysema on CT scanning can be enhanced by using specific data acquiring software programs, such as minimum intensity projection (MinIP) techniques [25]. Therefore, it is likely that CT analysis can be used to monitor the progression of emphysematous lung destruction and has the potential to serve as an imaging biomarker to assess the effect of therapeutics on emphysema [26]. Having said that, it is important to note that lung density measurements on CT can be affected by numerous factors such as patient size, depth of inspiration, the type of CT scanner used, collimation, and the reconstruction algorithm. Subjective assessment of bronchial wall thickening on HRCT scans is markedly influenced by window settings. Careful attention to synchronize the technical protocol is essential for comparing data among institutions and studies, and using the technique in multi-center clinical trials [27]. Despite the limitation, CT is the only readily accessible and relatively non-invasive technique that provides quantitative structure data *in vivo* and is the most promising biomarker for developing disease modifying drugs to treat COPD.

7.3.5 *Rheumatoid Arthritis*

Imaging biomarkers have played an important role in the development of disease modifying anti-rheumatic drugs (DMARDs). Outcomes measured by X-ray of the joints are the conventional regulatory approved end point to register drug products claiming inhibition of radiographic progression through a 1-year clinical study.

With the recent availability of effective biological DMARDs, new demands for imaging biomarkers have been created. Therapeutic strategy has shifted toward early, aggressive treatment before the onset of erosive joint damage in order to prevent irreversible functional disability. In this regard, MRI provides greater sensitivity to bone erosion than X-ray, especially in early RA when radiography is relatively uninformative. In addition, MRI has the ability to detect synovitis, joint effusion, and bone edema, which allows for identification of patients with aggressive phenotype of RA at a very early stage and evaluate response to therapy based on reduction in inflammation [28]. Therefore, MRI has the potential to serve as an endpoint in the assessment of structural damage, and imaging of inflammation may facilitate the identification of promising therapeutics in early development and potentially for dose optimization. More work is needed to assess if imaging of inflammation can be a successful surrogate marker in RA [29].

Ultrasound is another imaging modality that may prove utility as a biomarker of RA disease activity and progress. Inter-observe variability and lack of experience in multicenter clinical trials, however, limit its application in drug development [30].

In the preclinical context, significant data (e.g., micro-CT) have been accumulated in animal models to assess the efficacy on bone protection for DMARDs. The clinical translation for some of the cutting edge imaging technologies, such as PET of macrophages [31], has been limited by the fact that clinical outcome measures are sensitive to drug effects within the time frame of the clinical trial. Recent data however indicate that FDG-PET could be used to predict the clinical efficacy for RA patients treated with anti-tumor necrosis factor (TNF) agent [32].

7.3.6 *Osteoarthritis*

While tremendous efforts have been put toward the development of disease modifying osteoarthritis drugs (DMOADs), to date such efforts have been unsuccessful. Lack of appropriate biomarkers is the key factor for such failure. Currently, joint space narrowing (JSN) as determined by X-ray is the only surrogate endpoint for efficacy of a therapeutic intervention accepted by the regulatory agencies; however, its utility in clinical trials has presented significant challenges.

JSN has neither been shown to correlate with disease activity nor with abnormalities occurring relatively late in disease. Additionally, radiographic progress is too slow, and X-ray too imprecise, for the practical assessment of any therapeutic intervention. For a typical proof of concept trial for DMOADs, it has been estimated that more than 400 patients will be required for each arm, with greater than 1-year dosing needed to observe moderate efficacy.

Such limitations therefore necessitate large, long, and complex clinical trials for demonstration of efficacy. Such trials, however, still continue to fall short of establishing proof of efficacy. In fact, nine large clinical trials with DMOADs carried out over the last decade have all been unsuccessful. These failures underscore the need for identification and validation of additional biomarkers to monitor disease progression and to identify those patients most likely to progress. Therefore, a rapid surrogate marker (preferably between 3 to 6 months) for structural damage is critically needed. Currently, more sophisticated imaging modalities, such as MRI and molecular imaging, are being explored and adapted to overcome the limitations of standard X-ray [6].

Unlike X-ray, MRI can evaluate multiple pathological processes in OA, such as fragmentation and generation of articular cartilage, bone sclerosis, osteophytes, cyst formation, menisci and ligament structure, synovitis and bone marrow edema. MRI is the best imaging technique for noninvasive visualizing articular cartilage. It can also accurately measure cartilage thickness and volume, surface smoothness, as well as the distribution of disease changes [33]. Cartilage thinning as measured by MRI most closely resembles, and potentially more precisely reflects, JSN on X-ray. Bone marrow abnormality is another feature of OA that can be captured and measured by MRI. It has been associated with both pain and changes of certain biochemical biomarkers and can predict JSN and cartilage loss, especially at the area adjacent to the edema [34]. Furthermore, it is increasingly clear that early pathological changes are not captured well by X-ray but are usually evident on MRI. MRI also provides a method for noninvasive detection and quantification of biochemical changes in cartilage that precede morphologic deterioration.

In numerous clinical studies using cross sectional and longitudinal OA patient cohorts, MRI has shown adequate reliability, specificity, and sensitivity, as well as the ability to detect lesion progression within a reasonable observation time frame (1–2 years). This capacity, combined with the availability of robust imaging acquisition protocol for multi-center trials, indicate that MRI of cartilage has tremendous potential to be widely used in clinical trials for monitoring treatment response to structure modifying OA drugs.

Experience accumulated from ongoing and future studies will serve to solidify MRI of the cartilage as the preferred method of choice to obtain reliable and quantitative data on cartilage morphology [35]. With time, MRI of the cartilage may even serve as a surrogate marker for structure progression and clinical end point for DMOADs trials.

It should be pointed out, however, that MRI provides only limited information on cartilage quality beyond the surface of the disease loci; novel molecular imaging technologies will be needed to provide this additional information by assessing the molecular composition of cartilage. To date, the most commonly used modality for molecular imaging of cartilage has been T2 MRI. T2 is an MR relaxation time reflecting interactions between water molecules and between water and surrounding macromolecules, with increasing interaction leading to a decreased T2. So far, however, no relationship has been established between T2 changes and disease activity progression in clinical studies despite intense research for the last decade. This can be primarily attributed to the fact that T2 is affected by many physiological and pathological processes that relate to the state of cartilage. For example, physical activity is associated with MRI-based knee cartilage T2 measurements in asymptomatic subjects with and without OA risk factors [36].

In addition to T2, several other molecular imaging technologies have been the focus of attention in the field of OA biomarker development. Among them, T1 MRI (T1 in the rotating frame) and delayed gadolinium-enhanced magnetic resonance imaging (dGEMRIC) provide the most promise to potentially revolutionize OA biomarker development to fulfill the need to measure disease activity based on molecular mechanism and predict "rapid progressors" with precision [6].

7.4 Challenges for Clinical Translation and Optimization of Imaging Biomarkers

Despite their success so far and great future potential, imaging biomarkers have not been routinely incorporated into clinical trials and widely used as surrogate end points for drug product registration. There are numerous factors hindering the application of imaging biomarkers in clinical development. These challenges can be divided into three major categories, which I describe below.

7.4.1 *Financial and Logistic Issues*

Developing imaging biomarkers, especially target-specific probes for molecular imaging, is a costly and complex endeavor. As the cost of clinical development becomes prohibitively more expensive, the need for high quality biomarkers to reduce the overall cost and shorten the drug development timeline has become imperative, and thus the relative high cost of imaging is justified strategically. However, at the operational level, it is challenging to allocate resources to the development and implementation of imaging biomarkers in individual programs, especially within today's resource constrained environment. In particular, regulatory qualification of an imaging biomarker as a surrogate end point requires both substantial time and funding. Costs can be in the range of tens to hundreds of millions US dollar per approved surrogate end point. Therefore, collaboration between all stakeholders, such as the pharmaceutical industry, technology developers, academia, and regulatory agencies, is needed to share the cost for imaging biomarker development and ensure the technology is incorporated.

In addition to the cost factor, incorporating imaging biomarkers will increase the complexity for the execution of clinical trials. It will impact the study design, data documentation and reporting, study personnel education, and investigator site qualification and validation. It will likely restrict the site selection and extend the clinical study duration on most occasions.

7.4.2 *Technical Challenges*

Technology is the main driver for the development of novel imaging modalities and enhanced analysis algorithms. Great success has been made in utilizing cutting edge technologies in imaging biomarker development. However, more work in the following key areas is needed to optimize the current and develop the new imaging biomarkers: (1) increase resolution in 3D and time improves profiling of tissue, organ, and cells; (2) monitor images in more narrow time slices helps measure therapeutic effect with more precision; (3) develop new algorithms to enable data interpretation with more efficiency, and; (4) explore technique combination for the development of multi-modality platform.

In addition to the requirement for ever evolving technology advancement, there are two main prerequisites for the effective clinical translation of imaging biomarkers, which are standardization and validation.

Standardization concerns the acquisition parameters for imaging and the post-processing methods. They are essential steps to ensure reproducibility across different centers and apparatuses. They pose unique challenges for clinical translation of imaging biomarkers, which is not prominent at the preclinical stage. They include equipment evaluation, procedure standardization, data reproducibility and replication, inter-rater variability, the production and measurement of standards, inter-subject variance, choice of image reconstruction and segmentation algorithms, and automated versus observer-dependent image analysis [37]. Therefore, informatics is an integral component of this process. Approaches for informatics in the areas of controlled terminologies, image annotation, and image-processing algorithms will need to continue to evolve and mature with the expanding application of imaging biomarkers in clinical drug development. Advancement in this area requires collaboration among stakeholders through standardized data sharing in a secured environment through either third-party data brokers or open source approaches. Imaging societies, such as the Radiological Society of North America (RSNA), have taken steps in coordinating the standard establishment effort through its Quantitative Imaging Biomarker Alliance (QIBA). The group is a partnership between stakeholders from pharmaceutical and medical device manufacturers, imaging informatics companies, government agencies, imaging societies, and clinical research groups intend to develop and adopt hardware and software standards to achieve accurate and reproducible quantitative results from using imaging biomarkers. Such standardization initiatives and collaboration across the board will have a positive impact on the establishment of an integrated data sharing system among patient records, clinical research and outcome data, and promote personalized drug development and patient care.

The sensitivity, specificity, precision, and reproducibility of new biomarkers have to go through a rigorous validation process. The validation should be conducted in simulated models, animals, and humans. The changes in biomarker values should be correlated to the biological effect and clinical endpoints (qualification). The validation requirements are much higher for surrogate endpoints than for pharmacodynamic biomarkers. Qualification as a surrogate endpoint requires significant resources and will, in many cases, only be possible in a concerted collaborative effort by academia, industry, and regulatory authorities.

7.4.3 *Regulatory Hurdles*

Identification of therapeutic effects through validated surrogate endpoints can substitute for clinical end points, and the data obtained may be used as a primary end point in pivotal clinical trials for drug product registration. Qualification of surrogate imaging biomarkers requires the approval of regulatory authorities. Therefore, the involvement and alignment with regulatory agencies is critical for the future development and qualification of such biomarkers.

Accelerating the qualification process will require a collective effort among all relevant stakeholders. It remains a challenge to identify who will be the primary driver for this complex and expensive process. A well-defined regulatory approval process is needed to make the qualification possible. Considering the nature of the process, no single drug developer or academic center can complete the task. Therefore pre-competitive collaboration and partnership among stakeholders is required to obtain the necessary data. Biomarkers Consortium (http://www.biomarkersconsortium.org) is an example of this type of collaboration. It is a public–private partnership managed by the Foundation for the National Institutes of Health (NIH) in the USA [38]. Such a partnership has lead to the successful qualification of preclinical kidney toxicity biomarkers through the pilot FDA and European Medicines Agency (EMA) qualification process (http://www.emea.europa.eu/htms/human/mes/biomarkers.htm).

It remains to be seen if an imaging biomarker can be qualified through the same process. In order to make this happen, gaps need to be filled to address the most pressing issue, which is the need to establish standardized systems for the development, validation, qualification, and use of accurate, repeatable, and quantitative imaging biomarkers across instruments and settings. Publicly accessible data repositories for images, such as those from the Osteoarthritis Initiative (OAI), are of particular value to facilitate the process. OAI is a large NIH-funded multicenter longitudinal cohort study involving both academic centers and pharmaceutical companies, which has so far enabled the generation of large body of information on risk factors and biomarkers for the onset and progression of knee OA [36, 39]. Such efforts will undoubtedly accelerate the validation and qualification process for novel imaging biomarkers in clinical trials and drug development for OA. Another example comes from the field of oncology. The US FDA, National Cancer Institute (NCI), and Centers for Medicare and Medicaid Services (CMS) have initiated a collaborative effort to validate imaging biomarkers for clinical application through the Oncology Biomarker Quantification Initiative (OBQI). This features FDG-PET in predicting tumor response for non-Hodgkin's lymphoma and non-small cell lung cancer. In this initiative, the NCI develops validation protocols, and FDA provides guidance to encourage the use of imaging biomarkers to facilitate drug development for oncologic diseases.

7.5 Conclusions and Future Outlook

Despite the challenges, imaging biomarkers provide unique advantages over biochemical and other biomarkers in drug development. Tremendous progress has been made in translating the experience from preclinical development into the clinical development setting. Accelerated growth in the field is anticipated due to the rapid utilization of emerging novel technologies and maturation of the current platforms. Current available imaging biomarkers provide structural, physiological, and metabolic information. Novel imaging platforms come with great promise to annotate structure with molecular signatures that tightly link to the pathophysiology or to the therapeutic mechanism of actions. These cutting edge modalities will reveal information on *in vivo* pharmacokinetics, receptor expression and occupancy, and/or molecular signaling, which will greatly enhance the precision and effectiveness for modern drug research and development.

Emerging technologies will provide investigators with more powerful tools to develop imaging biomarkers to serve broad and yet specific needs. For instance, cyclotron becomes more affordable and easier to operate and maintain, which makes it feasible to have in-house PET facility for preclinical studies and in turn enhance the clinical translation further downstream. With more attention being paid to the development of biologics including monoclonal antibodies (mAbs) to treat various diseases, newly developed modalities such as immuno-PET will be more widely used to evaluate the *in vivo* behavior and efficacy of mAbs. It combines the high sensitivity and resolution of a PET camera with the precision of a mAb to carry out "comprehensive immunohistochemistry staining *in vivo*" [40]. Despite the tremendous upside, imaging biomarkers should not be considered a solution to all the challenges of drug development, and should not be used hastily or without full assessment of its pros and cons, as this will lead to incomplete and inaccurate results.

In addition, technology alone does not reflect the complex nature and the value of imaging biomarker development. The feasibility for clinical translation is the key to any initial assessment, as this reflects the true practical value of the new technology and platform. The primary driver for imaging biomarker development at the bedside resides in the need from patient care and clinical trials, and the capability of the imaging modality to fulfill the specific demand of drug development.

Lack of accepted imaging standards, variability in platforms across multiple sites, and limited data sharing due to divergent stakeholder priorities, continue to be the primary challenges for imaging biomarker clinical translation and development. More effort is needed to coordinate, conduct, and stimulate research and education about the development, standardization, validation, and qualification of imaging biomarkers. Such a task calls for more synchronized bench-to-bedside cooperation of radiologists, nuclear medicine specialists, clinicians, and basic scientists in physics, chemistry, biology, pathology, bioengineering, and bioinformatics.

Finally, considering that significant resources are needed to validate imaging biomarkers, public and private sector pre-competitive collaborations and partnerships are required. Proactive engagement with regulatory agencies will be critical to qualify a biomarker as a surrogate end point for clinical trials. Successful translation from bench-to-bedside through clinical development would reveal new insights and provide key lessons which may in turn promote future imaging biomarker development at the bench.

References

1. Hargreaves, R.J. (2008). The role of molecular imaging in drug discovery and development. *Clinical Pharmacology & Therapeutics*, **83**, pp. 349–353.
2. Alavi, A. and Reivich, M. (2002). Guest editorial: the conception of FDG-PET imaging, *Seminars in Nuclear Medicine*, **32**, pp. 2–5.
3. Deshpande, N., Foygel, K., Ren, Y., Rosenberg, J., and Willmann, J.K. (2011). Tumor angiogenic marker expression levels during tumor growth: longitudinal assessment with molecularly targeted microbubbles and US imaging, *Radiology*, **258**, pp. 804–811.
4. Choyke, P.L. (2011). Science to practice: angiogenic marker expression during tumor growth–can targeted US microbubbles help monitor molecular changes in the microvasculature?, *Radiology*, **258**, pp. 655–656.
5. Pysz, M.A., Gambhir, S.S., and Willmann, J.K. (2010). Molecular imaging: current status and emerging strategies, *Clinical Radiology*, **65**, pp. 500–516.
6. Parsons, S., Alesci, S., Feuerstein, G., and Wang, J. (2008). Biomarkers in the development of novel disease-modifying therapies for osteoarthritis, *Biomarkers in Medicine*, **2**, pp. 587–602.
7. Chandra, S., Carr, S., Muir, C., and Silva, M. (2005). Imaging biomarkers in drug development: an overview of opportunities and open issues, *Journal of Proteome Research* **4**, pp. 1134–1137.

8. Pien, H.H., Fischman, A.J., Sorensen, A.G., and Thrall, J.H. (2005). Using imaging biomarkers to accelerate drug development and clinical trials, *Drug Discovery Today*, **10**, pp. 259–266.
9. Rudin, M. (2009). Noninvasive structural, functional, and molecular imaging in drug development, *Current Opinion in Chemical Biology*, **13**, pp. 360–371.
10. Pincus, T. and Sokka, T. (2004). Quantitative measures and indices to assess rheumatoid arthritis in clinical trials and clinical care, *Rheumatic Disease Clinics of North America* **30**, pp. 725–751, vi.
11. van der Meel, R., Byrne, A.T., Gallagher, W.M., O'Connor, A.E., Oliveira, S., and Schiffelers, R.M. (2010). Recent advances in molecular imaging biomarkers in cancer: application of bench to bedside technologies, *Drug Discovery Today*, **15**, pp. 102–114.
12. O'Connor, J.P., Asselin, M.C., Buckley, D.L., Jackson, A., Jayson, G.C., and Parker, G.J. (2008). Quantitative imaging biomarkers in the clinical development of targeted therapeutics: current and future perspectives, *Lancet Oncology*, **9**, pp. 766–776.
13. Desar, I.M., Barentsz, J.O., Oyen, W.J. van der Graaf, W.T., van Herpen, C.M., and van Laarhoven, H.W. (2009). Beyond RECIST: molecular and functional imaging techniques for evaluation of response to targeted therapy, *Cancer Treatment Reviews*, **35**, pp. 309–321.
14. Morse, D.L. and Gillies, R.J. (2010). Molecular imaging and targeted therapies, *Biochemical Pharmacology*, **80**, pp. 731–738.
15. Brooks, D.J., and Pavese, N. (2011). Imaging biomarkers in Parkinson's disease, *Progress in Neurobiology,* Aug 30 95, pp. 614–628.
16. Sakoglu, U., *et al.* (2011). Paradigm shift in translational neuroimaging of CNS disorders, *Biochemical Pharmacology*, **81**, pp. 1374–1387.
17. Rinne, J. O., *et al.* (2010). 11C-PiB PET assessment of change in fibrillar amyloid-beta load in patients with Alzheimer's disease treated with bapineuzumab: a phase 2, double-blind, placebo-controlled, ascending-dose study, *Lancet Neurology*, **9**, pp. 363–372.
18. Chertkow, H. and Black, S. (2007). Imaging biomarkers and their role in dementia clinical trials, *Canadian Journal Neurological Sciences*, **34**(1), pp. S77– S83.
19. Hampel, H., Bokde, A.L., Prvulovic, D., and Teipel, S.J. (2011). Recent developments of functional magnetic resonance imaging research for drug development in Alzheimer's disease, *Progress in Neurobiolgy*, Jul 13 95, pp. 570–578.

20. de Lange, E.E., *et al.* (1999). Lung air spaces: MR imaging evaluation with hyperpolarized 3He gas, *Radiology,* **210**, pp. 851–857.
21. Samee, S., *et al.* (2003). Imaging the lungs in asthmatic patients by using hyperpolarized helium-3 magnetic resonance: assessment of response to methacholine and exercise challenge, *Journal of Allergy and Clinical Immunology*, **111**, pp. 1205–1211.
22. Muller, N.L. and Coxson, H. (2002). Chronic obstructive pulmonary disease. 4: imaging the lungs in patients with chronic obstructive pulmonary disease, *Thorax,* **57**, pp. 982–985.
23. Dirksen, A., *et al.* (1999). A randomized clinical trial of alpha(1)-antitrypsin augmentation therapy, *American Journal of Respiratory and Critical Care Medicine*, **160**, pp. 1468–1472.
24. Klein, J.S., Gamsu, G., Golden, J.A., Muller, N.L., and Webb, W.R. (1992). High-resolution CT diagnosis of emphysema in symptomatic patients with normal chest radiographs and isolated low diffusing capacity, *Radiology*, **182**, pp. 817–821.
25. Remy-Jardin, M., Copin, M.C., Duhamel, A., Gosselin, B., Remy, J., and Wurtz, A. (1996). Sliding thin slab, minimum intensity projection technique in the diagnosis of emphysema: histopathologic-CT correlation, *Radiology*, **200**, pp. 665–671.
26. de Jong, P.A., Coxson, H.O., Hogg, J.C., Long, F.R., Merkus, P.J. Tiddens, H.A., and Wong, J.C. (2006). Computed tomographic estimation of lung dimensions throughout the growth period, *European Respiratory Journal*, **27**, pp. 261–267.
27. Coxson, H.O. and Lam, S. (2009). Quantitative assessment of the airway wall using computed tomography and optical coherence tomography, *Proceedings of the American Thoracic Society*, **6**, pp. 439–443.
28. Peterfy, C.G. (2004). Is there a role for extremity magnetic resonance imaging in routine clinical management of rheumatoid arthritis?, *Journal of Rheumatology*, **31**, pp. 640–644.
29. Peterfy, C.G. (2004). MRI of the wrist in early rheumatoid arthritis, *Annals of the Rheumatic Diseases*, **63**, pp. 473–477.
30. Tesch, G., Amur, S., Bai, J.P., Lesko, L.J., Schousboe, J.T., and Siegel, J.N. (2010). Successes achieved and challenges ahead in translating biomarkers into clinical applications, *AAPS Journal*, **12**, pp. 243–253.
31. van der Laken, C.J., *et al.* (2008). Noninvasive imaging of macrophages in rheumatoid synovitis using 11C-(R)-PK11195 and positron emission tomography, *Arthritis & Rheumatism*, **58**, pp. 3350–3355.

32. Elzinga, E.H., *et al.* (2011). 18F-FDG PET as a tool to predict the clinical outcome of infliximab treatment of rheumatoid arthritis: an explorative study, *Journal of Nuclear Medicine*, **52**, pp. 77–80.
33. Burstein, D. and Gray, M. (2003). New MRI techniques for imaging cartilage, *Journal of Bone and Joint Surgery America*, **85**(A Suppl 2), pp. 70–77.
34. Eckstein, F., Cicuttini, F., Peterfy, C., Raynauld, J.P., and Waterton, J.C. (2006). Magnetic resonance imaging (MRI) of articular cartilage in knee osteoarthritis (OA): morphological assessment, *Osteoarthritis Cartilage*, **14**(Suppl A), pp. A46–A75.
35. Li, X., *et al.* (2007). *In vivo* T(1rho) and T(2) mapping of articular cartilage in osteoarthritis of the knee using 3 T MRI, *Osteoarthritis Cartilage*, **15**, pp. 789–797.
36. Hovis, K.K., *et al.* (2011). Physical activity is associated with magnetic resonance imaging-based knee cartilage T2 measurements in asymptomatic subjects with and those without osteoarthritis risk factors, *Arthritis & Rheumatism*, **63**, pp. 2248–2256.
37. Schuster, D.P. (2007). The opportunities and challenges of developing imaging biomarkers to study lung function and disease, *American Journal of Respiratory and Critical Care Medicine*, **176**, pp. 224–230.
38. Bai, J.P., *et al.* (2011). Translational biomarkers: from preclinical to clinical a report of 2009 AAPS/ACCP Biomarker Workshop, *AAPS Journal*, **13**, pp. 274–283.
39. Eckstein, F., Cotofana, S., Dreher, D., Frobell, R, John, M.R., Nevitt, M., and. Wirth, W. (2011). Greater rates of cartilage loss in painful knees than in pain-free knees after adjustment for radiographic disease stage: data from the osteoarthritis initiative, *Arthritis & Rheumatism*, **63**, pp. 2257–2267.
40. van Dongen, G.A. and Vosjan, M.J. (2010). Immuno-positron emission tomography: shedding light on clinical antibody therapy, *Cancer Biotherapy and Radiopharmaceuticals*, **25**, pp. 375–385.

Chapter 8

Translational Bioinformatics: Bridging the Biological and Clinical Divide

Indra Neil Sarkar

Center for Clinical and Translational Science, Department of Microbiology, College of Medicine, Department of Computer Science, College of Engineering and Mathematical Sciences, University of Vermont, Burlington, Vermont, USA

neil.sarkar@uvm.edu

8.1 Introduction

Thirty years since the first use of the term "bioinformatics" [1] the study of information related to life on earth has entered a new era. For much of the history of "bioinformatics" (which in this context is also used to refer to strongly related, although not necessarily synonymous terms such as "computational biology" or "biocomputing"), the attention has been on developing a deeper understanding of fundamental biology phenomena. Recent years have seen a new paradigm emerge for identifying relationships between molecular information and disease states, largely possible due to significant increases in the availability of biological and clinical data. The rapidly evolving field of translational bioinformatics (TBI) is core to

Translational Medicine: The Future of Therapy
Edited by James Mittra and Christopher-Paul Milne

ISBN 978-981-4316-99-6 (Hardback), 978-981-4364-84-3 (eBook)
www.panstanford.com

enabling the promise of unveiling such relationships. A major area of emphasis in TBI is the bridging between traditionally segregated biological and clinical knowledge sources, which has historically been the subject of domain-specific informatics communities. TBI aims to provide an integrative approach, which builds on focused domain-specific informatics approaches, toward the postulation of novel testable hypotheses [2].

While implicitly related to health, such as in the case of studying model organisms [3] or identifying molecular patterns in disease genes [4–6], only recently has there been specific attempts to develop TBI innovations to understand fundamental concepts in human disease and facilitate the identification of therapeutics or cures [7]. TBI focuses on developing hypotheses of the biological basis of human disease through "...the development of storage, analytic, and interpretive methods to optimize the transformation of increasingly voluminous biomedical data into proactive, predictive, preventative, and participatory health" [8]. To this end, TBI is the realization of biomedical informatics principles to develop linkages between the molecular processes of disease or dysfunction with phenotypic information (e.g., symptomatology), such as described in clinical sources.

The growth of TBI in recent years can also be attributed to significant advancements within both biological and clinical settings. In biology, we have seen the cost of sequencing the entire human genome (which cost approximately $3bn in 2001) plummet to mere thousands of dollars (with the promise of a $1000 genome in the not-too-distant future) [9]. In clinics, we are witnessing a revolution of informatics innovations being put into practice, such as electronic health record (EHR) systems in provider offices and health information exchange like never before imagined [10, 11]. Furthermore, and of equal importance, has been the development of participatory approaches to data gathering and analysis [12]. For example, we have seen the emergence of major consumer-driven genomics projects such as 23andMe [13] and the Genographic Project [14], which have contributed to increasing interest and thus expectations for genetic-based data to provide insights to our individual health and evolutionary history.

Together, the continual advances in both the clinical and biological realms are uniting to usher in a new era of medicine. Underpinning the success of integrating relevant data points that link biological data to clinical outcomes will be the innovations that come from the sub-domain of TBI. In many ways, TBI is still nascent in its demonstration of potential impact both for individuals as well as for entire populations. At the same time, TBI is built on fundamental principles of both bioinformatics and clinical informatics that have been maturing for more than three decades. This chapter puts TBI in the context of the rich history of bioinformatics and clinical informatics, and provides an overview of the approaches for linking across biological and clinical knowledge sources. Particular attention is given to approaches that enable the linking of biological and clinical data, especially as related to translational medicine.

8.2 A Genomic Revolution or Avalanche?

The promise of the Human Genome Project (HGP) was to provide a blueprint for developing a framework for understanding the molecular underpinning of disease and wellbeing [15]. The incremental advancements in our understanding of human health since the completion of the HGP has provided ample discussion about whether understanding the molecular blueprint for life will actually provide more insight than "tried and true," "back to the basic" biological and epidemiological studies [16]. However, the technology innovations that have emerged since the HGP have led to significant technological advances in sequence generation, assembly, and annotation (many of which were inspired by the HGP [17,18]). As the cost for sequencing entire genomes comes closer to $1000, the ability to acquire genomes for entire populations becomes conceivable. With the promotion of marker or Single Nucleotide Polymorphism (SNP)-based prediction of disease susceptibility (as offered by services such as 23andMe), the expectation of the general public may shift from "why would you want to sequence my genome?" to "why haven't you sequenced my genome?" While this notion suggests that there may be common good to be derived from sharing genomic data (e.g., through "crowdsourcing" [19]), it does introduce a new cadre of ethical and social issues [20]. Nonetheless, in the context of direct care there is increasing evidence that personal genomics will become an expectation in routine care [21], albeit with increased data security and informed consent procedures [22].

Thanks to carefully curated resources, such as the Online Mendelian Inheritance in Man (OMIM [23]), the biomedical research community has a long history of tracking gene–disease relationships. The advent of sequencing technologies increases the capability to study nucleotide or amino acid level patterns that can be associated with disease. Such studies have led to the concept of "Genome Wide Association Studies" (GWAS) [5]. GWAS aims to track mutations across many (or all) genes across populations with the goal to identify genes and gene mutations that may be associated with a phenotype of interest (e.g., disease status). Because the focus is on variations of DNA sequences (or SNP-based "haplotypes"), one does not need to sequence entire genomes. This has also resulted in major international initiatives ("HapMap") that focus on haplotype-based studies that can be used to facilitate the identification of disease-specific variation in DNA [24]. As sequencing technologies continue to improve, there is an increased ability to link genotypic variation to the often complex nature of disease.

Complementary to genomic data that are being generated for humans in pursuit of deeper understanding of genetic disorders, sequencing technologies have enabled unprecedented opportunities to sequence other organisms. At a minimum, the ability to have complete genotypic information for "model" organisms will help promote a deeper understanding of disease mechanisms in controlled environments [3]. At the other end of the spectrum, the capability to generate volumes of molecular sequence provides the opportunity to gain understanding of complex intra- and inter-organism relationships. For example, having a molecular understanding of vector–disease–host relationships may harbor valuable insights to understand zoonotic diseases that continue to plague the world [25].

Initially developed for gauging the biota of a particular biome, so called "metagenomic" approaches provide the facility to sample molecular sequence information across entire environments [26]. This approach to acquiring sequence data represents a significant advance in molecular sampling techniques, which traditionally have required the cultivation of clones before adequate DNA material could be collected for acquiring the molecular sequence. As such, the use of metagenomic approaches enables the acquisition of genetic information from organisms that are difficult to culture and thereby minimize the preparatory effort for environmental samples. In the context of human health, metagenomic technology has given rise to "microbiome" studies, which aim to provide a molecular sequence-based census of the microbes that live on or within us (where the human is the "environment"). A major goal of the NIH-led Human Microbiome Project [27] (along with the complementary EU MetaHIT [28]) is thus to identify linkages between microbiome populations and disease conditions (e.g., considering the microbial diversity in a person's gut relative to their susceptibility to colon cancer) [29].

Initiatives such as those described here have resulted in beyond-exponential growth of molecular sequence data in public (and private) repositories. For publicly accessible data, the International Sequence Data Consortium (INSDC) coordinates the deposition and availability of molecular sequence data [30]. Each of the individual repositories (GenBank in the United States, ENA in Europe, and DDBJ in Japan) for nucleotide sequence data enables access to a mirrored data set of all sequences deposited via publicly accessible Internet access points (e.g., via the Web or direct file transfer protocols). Each of the host organizations (the National Center for Biotechnology Information in the United States, the European Bioinformatics Institute, and the Center for Information Biology in Japan) have also developed and maintain browsing and analytic interfaces. Each of the organizations have devoted significant resources toward developing next generation approaches for both the data archiving and searching functionality that will continue to be needed by the biological and clinical communities and thus become one of the foundational components for TBI innovations.

Parallel to the growth in biological data has been the opportunity for developing new techniques for exploring and understanding the data that are generated. It is here that the majority of bioinformatics has been focused — in developing approaches to understand the complexity of biological information contained within repositories and to address data management tasks. The sheer volume of data available has in many ways reduced the need to generate primary data for hypothesis testing. The concept of an *in silico* hypothesis being generated solely from existing data is increasingly accepted by the biology community [31–33]. This is not to say that *in silico* approaches obviate the need for standard *in vitro* or *in vivo* validation; however, it does imply that *in silico* approaches might foster the development of testable hypotheses using standard approaches. The volume of data that is now available thus provides a rich substrate to develop potentially new paradigms for understanding biological processes, especially those associated with complex diseases.

8.3 The Clinical Data Deluge

Dating back to the middle of the twentieth century, there has been active research in developing computerized systems for maintaining clinical data associated with patient encounters [34]. Initially developed to facilitate patient care (such as those associated with direct care providers), clinical data capture systems have evolved to also have a significant database component [35]. Earlier systems predominantly focused on "read-only" views of relevant clinical data (e.g., laboratory results or transcribed dictation reports). Contemporary systems, termed as "electronic health record" systems, also allow for direct addition of information into clinical charts (e.g., orders via a "Computerized Provider Order Entry" (CPOE) system). In support of clinical care, there has been much research in the development of decision-support systems that can enable higher quality care [36]. For example, it is almost a standard feature for EHRs to have medication reconciliation and drug–drug interaction warning systems that can only be overridden by appropriate personnel.

Internationally, clinical care is mostly paper based [37]. In contrast to bioinformatics data repositories that are maintained by central and public resources (e.g., molecular sequence repositories are maintained and supported by public government funds), clinical data repositories and their associated EHR systems are installed and maintained by individual clinical enterprises (e.g., hospitals or private practices). Major initiatives, such as those associated with health care reform in the United States [38], strive to develop federated networks of clinical data, starting with ubiquitous deployment of EHR systems. These EHR systems would enable transfer of clinical data across "Health Information Exchange" (HIE) systems such that relevant information would be available to care providers for a given patient at the point of care, regardless of where the patient originates (e.g., necessary information, such as allergies, current medications, and immunizations about a patient from Massachusetts would be available to care providers if the patient was seen in an emergency department in California).

From a research perspective, the data captured within a clinical chart represent a rich set of data associated with a given individual. Aggregated according to defined criteria (e.g., individuals with a common set of diagnoses), patterns can be studied across entire populations. The biomedical informatics community is steadily working toward developing frameworks that will enable the sharing of clinical phenotype information such that they can be assembled into research data sets (e.g., the i2b2 project) [39]. There are of course a number of challenges, and thus research opportunities, from ethical, legal, and social perspectives (often collectively referred to as "ELSI" issues). From the very early days of the HGP, ELSI topics were considered a key element to enable the promise of genome-based diagnoses and treatments [15,40,41]. As TBI innovations usher in the potential to truly merge clinical and genomic data toward targeted diagnoses and treatments, either associated with research endeavors or during the course of routine clinical care, the ELSI issues can become magnified and are the subject of much discourse [42]. The resources associated with the HGP still provide an excellent primer on the issues to consider and have been updated to consider contemporary challenges [43].

Collectively, the volume of data that can be associated with an individual is immense. The myriad of laboratory results, signs and symptoms, problems, medications, and other clinically relevant data points provides the research community with great opportunities to identify patterns that may be associated with disease. Such heterogeneity of data types, each reflecting an important component of the disease or physiological phenotype of an individual, reflects a significant challenge in data integration across even a single individual, let alone across populations. The clinical informatics community has accordingly focused a great deal of attention on the development of standards and integration systems to begin addressing this challenge. There is still much room for innovation, and the promise of in-depth clinical data being captured for citizens around the globe will undoubtedly have significant implications for care and facilitate the development of new approaches for the betterment of human health.

8.4 Developing the Bridge Between Biological and Clinical Data

The ability to have the complete genome alongside clinical data for a given individual is a double-edged sword. On the one hand, having access to an entire genome together with comprehensive clinical data enables a new paradigm for genotype–phenotype correlations. On the other hand, the data deluge that will be generated may provide distracting or incomplete data relative to proven clinical prognostic markers (e.g., correlation between high HbA1C and diagnosis of Diabetes Mellitus). It is at this juxtaposition that the primary energy of TBI is focused [7]. Briefly stated, the fundamental goal of TBI is to develop testable hypotheses that provide clinical insights based on biological knowledge.

There are four major areas of emphasis in TBI [2] (Fig. 8.1). *Clinical genomics* is the integration of clinical and genomic information toward the development of genetic tests. Clinical genomics is perhaps one of the most classical forms of TBI, which is well known due to the popularity of gene tests like BRCA1 and BRCA2 mutations for breast cancer [44]. Clinical genomics approaches can include the stratification of populations based on genetic correlations, and thereby identify potential genes or mutations of clinical relevance (often using classical population genomics approaches). *Genomic medicine* is the direct linkage of health data

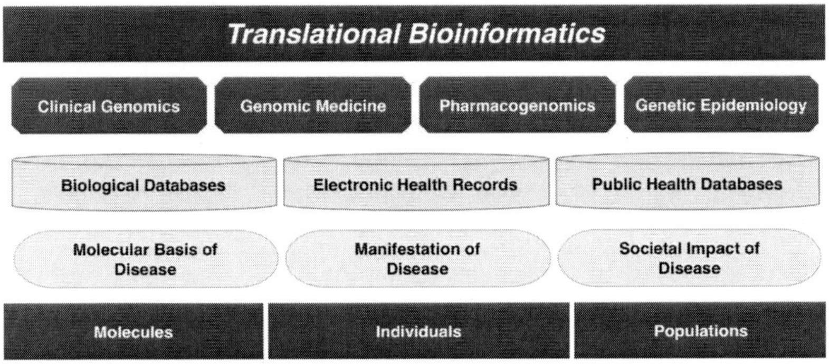

Figure 8.1 Translational bioinformatics overview. Translational Bioinformatics (TBI) involves the linkage of knowledge from molecules to individuals to populations. Building on core areas of bioinformatics (beveled rectangles: clinical genomics, genomic medicine, pharmacogenomics, and genetic epidemiology), TBI strives to integrate data from a range of heterogeneous data sources (cylinders) toward evaluating or developing new hypotheses that are associated with studying the molecular basis of, manifestation of, or societal impact of disease (ovals).

(such as captured in EHRs) with genomic information geared toward the understanding of the disease process. Building on population-level correlations that may have been identified from clinical genomic studies, genomic medicine inquiries strive to gain understanding of the molecular processes associated with disease etiology, and can be used for applications such as organizing diseases according to commonality of molecular features. Genomic medicine is often referred to as "Personalized Medicine," since suggested therapies can be personalized to the given genetic makeup of an individual (in contrast to generic approaches that have some non-specificity to an individual). *Pharmacogenomics* is the specific application of genomic medicine approaches to understand the complex relationships between drugs and genomes. The success of a pharmacogenomics inquiry will lead to the identification of a specific genomic target for a particular pharmacological substance. Subsequent understanding of the effect of this type of targeting can lead to the development of new drugs or adjustments to dosing of existing drugs. Perhaps the largest and most cited database of pharmacogenomic relationships is PharmGKB [45].

Finally, *genetic epidemiology* is the study of genomic patterns across populations using epidemiological methods. The motivation of genetic epidemiology is to develop preventive medical approaches that leverage genetic information for the betterment of public health. The United States' Centers for Disease Control and Prevention (CDC) coordinates the Human Genome Epidemiology Network (HuGENet), which links genomic studies with epidemiological information [46]. Studies such as the Framingham Heart Study are also incorporating GWAS approaches to help identify potential genomic targets that can be validated according to epidemiological information [47].

Clinical genomics, genomic medicine, pharmacogenomics, and genetic epidemiology are certainly not completely new disciplines [48]. The major challenge of TBI is thus not to develop new core tools in these areas. Instead, the focus of TBI is on how to build from the approaches and resources from each of these sub-disciplines to directly impact patient care. Perhaps the most important aspect of TBI is developing approaches to cross the space from research innovation to clinical intervention [49]. In translational medicine terminology, this is often referred to as the "T1" or "bench-to-bedside" translational barrier [49, 50]. The T1 translational barrier is specifically focused on understanding the molecular underpinnings of diseases in light of their clinical manifestations (in contrast to the "T2" translational barrier, which generally involves the translation of T1 findings into clinical practice). Conceptually, the premise is simple — develop a linkage between biological findings and develop a clinically relevant intervention for either the prevention or alteration of a disease state. In practice, it represents the holy grail of translational medicine [50].

The sheer volume of biological and clinical data means the TBI research community must develop a completely novel type of hypothesis — one that intrinsically links the deep biological underpinnings of disease with the complex phenotypes associated with the manifestation of disease. Biomedical researchers thus have in front of them a challenge akin to the one given to rocket scientists and physicists in the 1960s to put a man on the moon. However, the heterogeneity of the data as it is currently available — from file formats to standards for representation — suggests that it would be a challenge to even decipher the knowledge that is currently embodied in the collective knowledge source of biology and medicine. A major challenge that the TBI community needs to address is the integration of existing knowledge across a trans-disciplinary array of clinical genomics, genomic medicine, pharmacogenomics, and genetic epidemiology sources. Each of these sub-communities has evolved relatively independently of each other, resulting in specific precisions in terminology that are specific to each community. Some of this challenge may be addressed using "ontologies," a computer readable construct for representing knowledge [51,52]. Building on the success of projects such as the Gene Ontology (GO) [53,54]) and International Classification of Diseases (ICD) [55], there is some hope to systematically represent knowledge within a given resource. Since the mid 1980s there have been concerted efforts to develop linkages between knowledge representation standards such as ontologies. The Unified Medical Language System (UMLS) [56], developed and maintained by the United States National Library of Medicine, is a collection of over 100 such knowledge representation standards, including ones such as ICD and GO.

Through the use of knowledge representation standards, one can start to develop linkages between knowledge sources [57,58]. Because different knowledge sources may use different knowledge representation standards to represent the same concept, some effort must often be given to the process of "semantic harmonization." Sometimes semantic harmonization is required even if two knowledge sources are using the same knowledge representation standard, but have different interpretations of how the standard should be applied. Entire consortia have developed around the development, use, and maintenance of knowledge representation standards. Many of the decisions about harmonization require endorsement by such consortia. Within the health care community, the Systematized Nomenclature of Medicine–Clinical Terms (SNOMED CT) [59] is rapidly becoming the accepted standard for representing clinical information, especially for the purposes of integrating clinical data from multiple sources. SNOMED CT is maintained by the International Health Terminology Standards Development Organization (IHTSDO) [60], and endorsed by major governments, including the United States and those in the European Union.

The use of knowledge representation standards makes data accessible to computers (what is often termed "machine readable"). This is becoming an increasingly necessary process, since the volume of data that would need to be processed and analyzed is simply too much for manual review. Also, the complexity of relationships that may exist in even a single knowledge source might be better traversed using computational approaches. Approaches that leverage knowledge representation standards are referred to as "semantic." The Semantic Web (SW) accordingly represents the science for leveraging semantic relationships between atoms of knowledge, with an ultimate goal for new knowledge to be identified through the semantic linkages [61].

A core aspect of TBI is built on the ability to semantically link knowledge between biological foundations and clinical scenarios. While the principles and theories of SW-based approaches have been described and proven in controlled environments, there remain great challenges for the realization of a truly linked environment that can bridge biological and clinical data. Perhaps the biggest challenge is the development of approaches for systematically representing knowledge using common knowledge representation standards. Amidst the number of ontologies and controlled vocabularies that have been developed in both the biological and clinical communities, there is still limited adoption to the level whereby SW approaches can truly be leveraged. This is not indicative of researchers or data creators being unaware or hesitant to make use of knowledge representation standards. Instead, there are significant barriers to determining which standards to use, or how to implement the standards.

The choice and implementation of a given standard depends greatly on the types of data that are being represented. Within the clinical realm, the most used standards are those that are associated with billing (which is thus directly tied to the financial system used to pay for services). Similarly, in the biological realm, the standards that have achieved highest rates of adoption are those tied to publication or data submission requirements. Major standards bodies exist for both the biological (e.g., the Genome Standards Consortium (GSC) [62]) and clinical (e.g., Health Level 7 (HL7) [63]) domains that strive to directly address the need for increased standards development and adoption. In a trans-disciplinary situation, such as faced by the TBI community, there are limited ontologies that can be used to uniformly represent knowledge across the full spectrum of biomedicine. Indeed, the scope to develop such a comprehensive ontology would be a significant endeavor in itself. There is established work toward developing ontologies for representing a wide array of knowledge (e.g., SUMO [64] or DOLCE [65]); however, there has been a minimal concerted effort to date for developing such an integrative ontology specifically for biomedicine.

Equally challenging is the availability of a uniform representation (using any standard) of information within biological and clinical knowledge stores that contain legacy data. As the volume of both biological and clinical data being generated increase, the volume of "legacy" data is proportionally increasing. While standards may be adopted for contemporary and future studies, the linkage to these legacy data can be an essential aspect of translational inquiries. Entire centers have been established (e.g., the National Center for Biomedical Ontology (NCBO) at Stanford University [66]) to facilitate the access and browsing of available knowledge representation standards (through the NCBO BioPortal [67]) and providing Web-based services (NCBO Annotator [68]) that enable the annotation of data with knowledge representation standards. These types of services complement resources such as the UMLS and its associated MetaMap annotation tool [69], which can both be accessed and downloaded with a free license from the National Library of Medicine. Systems like NCBO Annotator and MetaMap are examples of "Natural Language Processing" (NLP) systems. NLP is a significant area of research across the biomedical informatics spectrum, with the key goal to transform natural language (e.g., either text or voice) into a form that can be readily incorporated into computer systems [70–73]. Nearly every knowledge base associated with either biological or clinical data has some data that would be made better accessible for computability through the use of some NLP approach.

Notwithstanding the challenges of representing biological and clinical knowledge, the biggest challenge that is faced by TBI is *how to develop linkages*. Knowledge representation standards thus represent a key infrastructural step, in addition to other components such as efficient parallel computing environments, adequate storage space, and meaningful visualization of data and subsequent inferences made for data analyses. Within both the biological and clinical realms there has been significant research energy in analyzing and interpreting data within constrained contexts. TBI requires something much greater. TBI requires the development of methodologies and approaches that can truly interpret fundamental biological data in the context of clinical scenarios. The expansion of computational approaches that incorporates a wide array of data types, can interpret a myriad of seemingly unrelated concepts, and still provide clinically meaningful testable hypotheses, is a significant undertaking. The success of TBI will thus be the amalgam of trans-disciplinary knowledge and approaches to analyze and integrate biological and clinical data.

8.5 A Look at the Future

The biomedical enterprise is at the cusp of uncovering unprecedented insights into the etiology of disease and developing an array of therapeutic approaches that have until now been topics of science fiction. For more than three decades, the biological and clinical realms of informatics have worked to develop a suite of innovations that provide the substrate wherefrom TBI is emerging. As the volume of data being generated in the biological and clinical arenas continues to exceed exponentially, there will be increasing need to develop informatics approaches for handling the data deluge. For biological data sets, it will continue to be essential to uncover underpinning phenomena associated with life functions (or, in the case of disease, dysfunction). Similarly, the availability of clinical data will be expected to provide new innovations for delivering higher quality care at reduced costs. Simultaneously, the TBI community will seek to develop new approaches to linking fundamental biological phenomena with health care outcomes.

The success of translational medicine depends on the assembly of trans-disciplinary teams that collectively span the major areas of concentration in TBI, consisting minimally of biologists,

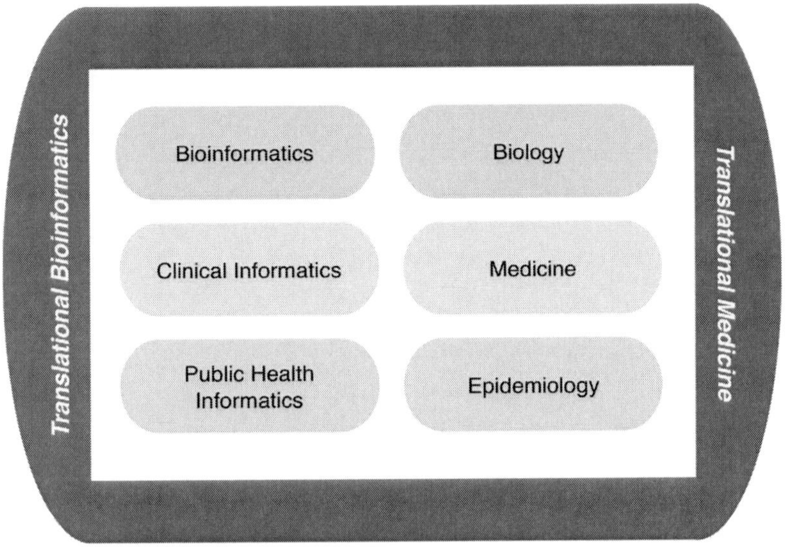

Figure 8.2 Translational bioinformatics as it relates to translational medicine. As translational medicine involves integration of knowledge across biology, medicine, and epidemiology, translational bioinformatics will require the integration of approaches from bioinformatics, clinical informatics, and public health informatics.

clinicians, and epidemiologists [49,50]. "Bioinformaticians," "clinical informaticians," and "public health informaticians" respectively work with each of these constituencies to support analyses and develop new hypotheses. The TBI community therefore consists of informaticians that aim to integrate the methodologies and insights across the spectrum of biomedicine (Fig. 8.2). As translational medicine continues to mature and trans-disciplinary teams are assembled, there will be an increased need for TBI specialists. The currently limited number of informaticians in each of the domain-specific areas will only be further highlighted by this growing need. Training programs and curricula that incorporate TBI concepts will accordingly become more essential to achieve many of the promises of translational medicine. An essential step will thus be the promotion of forums where TBI innovations can be shared across the range of domains associated with translational medicine (e.g., the AMIA Summit on Translational Bioinformatics).

Looking back to the completion of the HGP or the advent of the EHR, it would have been difficult to imagine how such seemingly separate endeavors would become intertwined in guiding the future of medicine. Yet, we are now in the midst of discussions of how Genome Wide Association Studies can be used to guide the next discoveries given volumes of clinical data. Already, we have started to see pioneering projects emerge such as the NIH-funded eMERGE (Electronic Medical Records and GEnomics) network [74], where the potential of linking clinical data (associated with individuals with specific conditions) and genomic data (from GWAS) is being explored across five sites (University of Washington/Hutchinson Cancer Center, Marshfield Clinic, Mayo Clinic, Northwestern University, and Vanderbilt University). The infrastructure and validation of findings from such projects will be essential for the success of future TBI endeavors.

As has been demonstrated in the last decade, the volume of data being generated will continue to exceed exponential growth. This suggests that the future of TBI will depend not only on the development of new approaches for linking heterogeneous data types, but also on managing unprecedented amounts of data (far exceeding any previous notion of "looking for a needle in a haystack"). TBI will undoubtedly be essential for crossing the translational barrier from bench to bedside. As this chapter has emphasized, a key step toward this crossing will be the development of linkages between biological and clinical data types. Through these linkages, the individual hypotheses that are generated within biological or clinical silos can be assembled into truly paradigm shifting hypotheses that may usher in a new era of medicine — one where translational medicine is the norm, not a dream of the future.

8.6 Concluding Remarks

Nearly a decade since the completion of the HGP, the biomedical enterprise is faced with the question of whether genomic data might actually play an important role in the care of patients. The field of TBI has evolved from traditional bioinformatics to specifically focus on the development of the necessary innovations for linking the biological and clinical realms. The translation of biological insights such that they may be used in light of clinical practice is certainly not new; however, in light of advancements in genomic acquisition technologies, the sheer volume of data requires a new paradigm for analysis and clinical interpretation. TBI aims to provide a trans-disciplinary framework, built on informatics innovations across the entire spectrum of biomedicine, which may help unveil basic biological insights that can be corroborated with clinical knowledge. In addition to the direct challenges that are faced by the TBI community (such as those associated with heterogeneous data integration), the practical challenges are also great (e.g., as associated with the ethical, legal, and social implications). In surmounting these challenges, the trans-disciplinary approach that is germane to TBI has the potential to provide the necessary innovations to cross the chasm between the biological insights and clinical impact.

References

1. Hogeweg, P., and Hesper, B. (1978). Interactive instruction on population interactions. *Computational Biology and Medicine* **8,** pp. 319–327.
2. Sarkar, I.N., *et al.* (2011). Translational bioinformatics: linking knowledge across biological and clinical realms. *Journal of the American Medical Informatics Association: JAMIA* **18**(4), pp. 354–357.
3. Muller, B., and Grossniklaus, U. (2010). Model organisms–A historical perspective. *Proteomics* **73**(11), pp. 2054–2063.
4. Moore, J.H. (2010). Detecting, characterizing, and interpreting nonlinear gene-gene interactions using multifactor dimensionality reduction. *Advances in Genetics.* **72**, pp. 101–116.
5. Manolio, T.A. (2010). Genomewide association studies and assessment of the risk of disease. *New England Journal of Medicine* **363**(2), pp. 166–176.
6. Rannala, B. (2001). Finding genes influencing susceptibility to complex diseases in the post-genome era. *American Journal of PharmacoGenomics* **1**(3), pp. 203–221.
7. Butte, A.J. (2008). Translational bioinformatics: coming of age. *Journal of the American Medical Informatics Association* **15**(6), pp. 709–714.

8. *American Medical Informatics Association (AMIA) Strategic Plan* (2006). [cited 2011 January 10, 2011]; Available from: http://www.amia.org/inside/stratplan.
9. Wolinsky, H. (2007). The thousand-dollar genome. Genetic brinkmanship or personalized medicine? *EMBO Report* **8**(10), pp. 900–903.
10. Vest, J.R., *et al.* (2011). Factors motivating and affecting health information exchange usage. *Journal of the American Medical Informatics Association* 18, pp. 143–149.
11. Wright, A., *et al.* (2010). Physician attitudes toward health information exchange: results of a statewide survey. *Journal of the American Medical Informatics Association* **17**(1), pp. 66–70.
12. Eriksson, N., *et al.* (2010). Web-based, participant-driven studies yield novel genetic associations for common traits. *PLoS Genet* **6**(6), p. e1000993.
13. https://www.23andme.com/.
14. https://genographic.nationalgeographic.com/genographic/index.html.
15. Watson, J.D. (1990). The human genome project: past, present, and future. *Science* **248**(4951), pp. 44–49.
16. Justman, M., Bezold, C., and Rowley, W. (2002). Genomics and society: four scenarios for 2015. *Foresight* **4**(4), pp. 29–36.
17. Metzker, M.L. (2010). Sequencing technologies — the next generation. *Nature Reviews Genetics* **11**(1), pp. 31–46.
18. Horner, D.S., *et al.* (2010). Bioinformatics approaches for genomics and post genomics applications of next-generation sequencing. *Brief Bioinform* **11**(2), pp. 181–197.
19. Prainsack, B., and Wolinsky, H. (2010). Direct-to-consumer genome testing: opportunities for pharmacogenomics research? *Pharmacogenomics* **11**(5), pp. 651–655.
20. Vijverberg, S.J., Cornel, M.C., and Pieters, T. (2010). Ethical and social issues in pharmacogenomics testing. *Current Pharmaceutical Design* **16**(2), pp. 245–252.
21. Gollust, S.E., *et al.* (2011). Motivations and perceptions of early adopters of personalized genomics: Perspectives from Research Participants. *Public Health Genomics* 15(1), pp. 22–30.
22. Haga, S.B., and O'Daniel, J. (2011). Public Perspectives Regarding Data-Sharing Practices in Genomics Research. *Public Health Genomics* 14(6), pp. 319–324.

23. Amberger, J., *et al.* (2009). McKusick's Online Mendelian Inheritance in Man (OMIM). *Nucleic Acids Research* **37** (Database issue), pp. D793–D796.
24. Manolio, T.A., and Collins, F.S. (2009). The HapMap and genome-wide association studies in diagnosis and therapy. *Annual Review of Medicine* **60**, pp. 443–456.
25. Haagmans, B.L., Andeweg, A.C., and Osterhaus, A.D. (2009). The application of genomics to emerging zoonotic viral diseases. *PLoS Pathogens.* **5**(10), pp. e1000557.
26. Chistoserdova, L. (2010). Recent progress and new challenges in metagenomics for biotechnology. *Biotechnology Letters* **32**(10), pp. 1351–1359.
27. http://commonfund.nih.gov/hmp/overview.aspx.
28. http://www.metahit.eu/.
29. Hattori, M., and Taylor, T.D. (2009). The human intestinal microbiome: a new frontier of human biology. *DNA Research* **16**(1), pp. 1–12.
30. Cochrane, G., Karsch-Mizrachi, I., and Nakamura, Y. (2011). The International Nucleotide Sequence Database Collaboration. *Nucleic Acids Research* **39**(Database issue), pp. D15–D18.
31. Deisboeck, T.S., *et al.* (2009). *In silico* cancer modeling: is it ready for prime time? *Nature Clinical Practice Oncology* **6**(1), pp. 34–42.
32. Kollmann, M., and Sourjik, V. (2007). *In silico* biology: from simulation to understanding. *Current Biology* **17**(4), pp. R132–R134.
33. Di Ventura, B., *et al.* (2006). From *in vivo* to *in silico* biology and back. *Nature* **443**(7111), pp. 527–533.
34. Greenes, R.A., *et al.* (1969). Design and implementation of a clinical data management system. *Computers and Biomedical Research* **2**(5), pp. 469–485.
35. Staggers, N., Snyder-Halpern, R., and Thompson, C.B. (2001). History and trends in clinical information systems in the United States. *Journal of Nursing Scholarship* **33**(1), pp. 75–81.
36. Sim, I., *et al.* (2001). Clinical decision support systems for the practice of evidence-based medicine. *Journal of the American Medical Informatics Association* **8**(6), pp. 527–534.
37. Williams, F., and Boren, S.A. (2008). The role of the electronic medical record (EMR) in care delivery development in developing countries: a systematic review. *Informatics in Primary Care* **16**(2), pp. 139–145.

38. Health information technology: initial set of standards, implementation specifications, and certification criteria for electronic health record technology (2010). Final rule. *Federal Register* **75**(144), pp. 44589–44654.
39. Weber, G.M., *et al.* (2009). The Shared Health Research Information Network (SHRINE): a prototype federated query tool for clinical data repositories. *Journal of the American Medical Informatics Association* **16**(5), pp. 624–630.
40. Jin, J. (2000). An evaluation of the Ethical, Legal and Social Implications program of the U.S. Human Genome Project. *Princeton Journal of Bioethics* **3**(1), pp. 35–50.
41. Meslin, E.M., Boyer, J.T., and Thomson, E.J. (1997). The Ethical, Legal, and Social Implications Research Program at the National Human Genome Research Institute. *Kennedy Institute of Ethics Journal* **7**(3), pp. 291–298.
42. Oliver, J.M., and McGuire, A.L. (2011) Exploring the ELSI universe: critical issues in the evolution of human genomic research. *Genome Medicine* **3**(6), pp. 38.
43. http://www.ornl.gov/sci/techresources/Human_Genome/elsi/elsi .shtml.
44. Neuhausen, S.L., and Ostrander, E.A. (1997). Mutation testing of early-onset breast cancer genes BRCA1 and BRCA2. *Genetic Testing* **1**(2), pp. 75–83.
45. Thorn, C.F., Altman, R.B., and Klein, T.E. (2005). PharmGKB: the pharmacogenetics and pharmacogenomics knowledge base. *Methods in Molecular Biology* **311**, pp. 179–191.
46. Little, J., and Hawken, S. (2010). On track? Using the Human Genome Epidemiology Roadmap. *Public Health Genomics* **13**(4), pp. 256–266.
47. Ma, L., *et al.* (2010). Genome-wide association analysis of total cholesterol and high-density lipoprotein cholesterol levels using the Framingham heart study data. *BMC Medical Genetics* **11**, pp. 55.
48. Martin-Sanchez, F., *et al.* (2004). Synergy between medical informatics and bioinformatics: facilitating genomic medicine for future health care. *Journal of Biomedical Informatics* **37**(1), pp. 30–42.
49. Sarkar, I.N. (2010). Biomedical informatics and translational medicine. *Journal of Translational Medicine* **8**, pp. 22 doi:10.1186/1479-5876-8-22.
50. Woolf, S.H. (2008). The meaning of translational research and why it matters. *JAMA* **299**(2), pp. 211–213.

51. Blake, J. (2004). Bio-ontologies-fast and furious. *Nature Biotechnology* **22**(6), pp. 773–774.
52. Rubin, D.L., Noy, N.F., and Shah, N.H. (2008). Biomedical ontologies: a functional perspective. *Briefings in Bioinformatics* **9**(1), pp. 75–90.
53. Ashburner, M., and Lewis, S. (2002) On ontologies for biologists: the Gene Ontology–untangling the web. *Novartis Foundation Symposium*. **247**, pp. 66–80; discussion 80–83, 84–90, 244–252.
54. http://www.geneontology.org.
55. http://www.who.int/classifications/icd/en/.
56. Bodenreider, O. (2004). The Unified Medical Language System (UMLS): integrating biomedical terminology. *Nucleic Acids Research* **32** (Database issue), pp. D267– D270.
57. Cantor, M.N., *et al.* (2005). Genestrace: phenomic knowledge discovery via structured terminology. *Pacific Symposium on Biocomputing*, pp. 103–114.
58. Sam, L.T., *et al.* (2009). PhenoGO: an integrated resource for the multiscale mining of clinical and biological data. *BMC Bioinformatics* **10**(l,2), pp. S8, doi:10.1186/1471-2105-10-S2-S8.
59. http://www.ihtsdo.org/snomed-ct/.
60. http://www.ihtsdo.org/.
61. Ruttenberg, A., *et al.* (2007). Advancing translational research with the Semantic Web. *BMC Bioinformatics* **8**(3), pp. S2 doi:10.1186/1471-2105-8-S3-S2.
62. http://gensc.org/gc_wiki/index.php/Main_Page.
63. http://www.hl7.org/.
64. Niles, I., and Pease, A. (2001). Towards a standard upper ontology. *Proceedings of the international conference on Formal Ontology in Information Systems*, 2001, pp. 2–9.
65. Gangemi, A., *et al.* (2003). Sweetening WORDNET with DOLCE. *AI Magazine* **24**(2), pp. 13–24.
66. http://www.bioontology.org/.
67. http://bioportal.bioontology.org/.
68. Shah, N.H., *et al.* (2009). Comparison of concept recognizers for building the open Biomedical Annotator. *BMC Bioinformatics* **10**(9), pp. S14, doi:10.1186/1471-2105-10-S9-S14.
69. Aronson, A.R. (2001). Effective mapping of biomedical text to the UMLS Metathesaurus: the MetaMap program. *Proceedings of AMIA Symposium*, pp. 17–21.

70. Meystre, S.M., *et al.* (2008). Extracting information from textual documents in the electronic health record: a review of recent research. *Yearbook of Medical Informatics*, pp. 128–144.

71. Raja, U., *et al.* (2008). Text mining in healthcare. Applications and opportunities. *Journal of Healthcare Information Management* **22**(3), pp. 52–56.

72. Ananiadou, S., Kell, D.B., and Tsujii, J. (2006). Text mining and its potential applications in systems biology. *Trends in Biotechnology* **24**(12), pp. 571–579.

73. Shatkay, H. (2005). Hairpins in bookstacks: information retrieval from biomedical text. *Briefings in Bioinformatics* **6**(3), pp. 222–238.

74. *https://*http://www.mc.vanderbilt.edu/victr/dcc/projects/acc/index.php/Main_Page.

Part 4

Institutional Dynamics of Translational Medicine

Chapter 9

Exploiting Translational Medicine Through Public–Private Partnerships: A Case Study of Scotland's Translational Medicine Research Collaboration

James Mittra
ESRC Innogen Centre and Science, Technology and Innovation Studies (STIS), University of Edinburgh, Old Surgeons' Hall, High School Yards, Edinburgh EH1 1LZ, UK
james.mittra@ed.ac.uk

9.1 Introduction and Background

The pharmaceutical industry continues to face a number of significant challenges to its conventional R&D model and commercial strategies. There is a high attrition rate of compounds in phase 2 clinical trials; the gap between drug discovery and development is hindering innovation and the speed of compounds through the development pathway; companies are more than ever reliant on externally sourced knowledge and expertise in life science; and better access to patients and tissue samples is needed to exploit new methods to improve the safety and efficacy profiles of therapies

Translational Medicine: The Future of Therapy
Edited by James Mittra and Christopher-Paul Milne

ISBN 978-981-4316-99-6 (Hardback), 978-981-4364-84-3 (eBook)
www.panstanford.com

[1]. Furthermore, a significant and often ignored challenge is what might be termed the "problem of maturity"; that is, drugs have already been developed for the easy targets and now that they are off-patent, they no longer attract the high profit margins necessary for sustainable growth [2]. In response to these challenges of sustainable innovation, amongst many others, large pharmaceutical firms have, in addition to recurrent waves of merger, acquisition, and strategic alliance behaviour [3,1], embraced the concept and underlying principles of translational medicine (TM) and entered a new experimental phase as they test different commercial and R&D models and strategic options. In particular, firms have sought to exploit interdisciplinary and collaborative research to complement in-house R&D and enable them to better access new science and technology and plug some of the translational gaps that threaten to undermine the conventional pharmaceutical business model that has predominated for decades. One key trend has been the development of public–private partnerships to facilitate the translation of novel compounds from bench to bedside. Such models require that a number of different organizations, often with diverse agendas, goals, and expectations, work together and share knowledge, resources, and expertise to improve the success rate of drug discovery and development.

TM offers the pharmaceutical industry a potential mechanism through which to exploit closer interaction between R&D and clinical development groups both within the firm, and between the commercial and academic/public sector. Industry anticipates that the successful implementation of TM processes, mechanisms, and strategies will help it to improve drug discovery and development, and perhaps ultimately contribute to resolving the problem of innovation deficit and low productivity within the sector. The expectation is that TM will, at the very least, help reduce attrition of compounds in phase 2, as well as contribute to improvements in the safety and efficacy of new treatments; thus meeting the increasingly strict requirements of regulatory agencies.

This chapter provides an analysis of a public/private TM initiative that was established in Scotland in 2006. The data that inform this case study come from 20 semi-structured interviews conducted with scientists, managers, clinicians, and other key stakeholders directly involved in the Translational Medicine Research Collaboration (TMRC), and/or with key roles in contributing to the UK's broader TM strategy. It also draws on substantial primary and secondary data collected on the evolution and dynamics of the pharmaceutical industry (including interviews with senior R&D managers and scientists at five top global pharmaceutical companies); conducted as part of the Economic and Social Research Council (ESRC) funded Innogen Centre's research program at the University of Edinburgh. The case study also draws on documents the TMRC released in the public domain (including press releases) during the early stages of the collaboration.

The TMRC was a broad-based collaboration focused on the identification and validation of new biomarkers relevant to commercial drug development. It serves as an example of a promising collaborative project with a high degree of institutional buy-in that appeared capable of tackling a number of translational challenges, as well as promising broader commercial and public health benefits. However, it also serves as a cautionary tale about the capricious and uncertain commercial environment for biopharmaceutical R&D, where external factors and the emergence of new strategic priorities can threaten the future of such initiatives. In this case, the takeover of the lead pharmaceutical firm Wyeth by its rival Pfizer led to the eventual collapse of the collaboration after the first 5-year round of funding ended. However, there were other challenges with the operational structure and strategic scope of the partnership that also need to be addressed. This case study offers many good lessons and insights about the institutional infrastructures and organizational relationships that need to be nurtured and made to work if TM is to fulfil its promise of improving healthcare innovation and meeting the diverse needs of key stakeholders. It also has important implications for industry-driven TM initiatives, where participating stakeholders may not have the same basic expectations and institutional goals. These key lessons will be drawn out in this chapter through an account of the rise and eventual collapse of the TMRC.

9.2 History and Background to TMRC

The TMRC was formally established on 1 April 2006 with the principal aim to develop and exploit a world leading network of clinical and scientific excellence in Scotland, and make significant contributions to the discovery, development, and delivery of new diagnostics and therapeutics [1]. Described at the time, both in the press and by key interview informants, as the first large-scale collaboration between industry, government, and academia, the Initiative received initial funding of $50 million for 5 years of research during April 2006–2011. The collaboration involved the medical schools of four of Scotland's leading research universities (Aberdeen, Dundee, Edinburgh, and Glasgow); the associated cities' health boards; Scotland's economic development agency (Scottish Enterprise); and the global pharmaceutical firm Wyeth. Scottish Enterprise's vision for a major life science collaboration in Scotland (to generate revenue, jobs, and inward investment) coincided with Wyeth's interest in developing a public–private partnership around TM, which it had initially tried to do in the United States. The idea was to set up a translational initiative beyond the preclinical phase, and TMRC was born out of this shared desire and commitment to invest by Wyeth and Scottish Enterprise.

A proclaimed institutional goal of the TMRC was the discovery and validation of biomarkers for the diagnosis and monitoring of human disease. The reason for organizing the collaboration as a public–private initiative was recognition that successful life science innovation requires institutionally diverse knowledge, resources and expertise as well as appropriate networks of professionals to bridge translational gaps [4]. All the interview respondents made explicit reference to the importance of interdisciplinary teams and new institutional partnerships as a key requirement for a successful translational strategy. Scotland's reputation in life science innovation and strong clinical and research infrastructure made it the location of choice for Wyeth's decision-makers [5], although one cannot discount the additional pull factor of Scottish Enterprise's commitment to jointly fund the initiative. Wyeth clearly wanted to exploit the potential of TM, particularly in the field of biomarker research, to facilitate in-house decisions about whether or not to progress phase 2 compounds.

TMRC involved the establishment of a core research laboratory linked to four major academic centres; as well as four NHS Trusts and Scotland's Clinical Research Network. The basic underlying philosophy was to creatively combine the resources and expertise of the key stakeholders to successfully complete approximately 100 TM projects in the first 5 years of funding, with the expectation that the collaboration would continue with additional funding for a further 5 years. It was intended that most of the individual projects would focus on basic research, but some would involve specific work on compounds supplied by Wyeth from their existing product pipeline.

9.3 Organizational Structure of the Initiative

Wyeth and Scottish Enterprise were the two principal sponsors of TMRC. Each committed core funding for the first 5 years of the Initiative (Wyeth committed $53.5m and Scottish Enterprise $33m). Scottish Enterprise's role was to be both an investor and facilitator of the initiative, with Wyeth taking on a more active role as both sponsor and driver of specific TM activities. Wyeth had already been one of the first-movers within industry to pursue a TM strategy, for example in adopting translational approaches to biomarker discovery and transcriptional profiling. Through this investment, Wyeth hoped to be able to leverage and exploit these new institutional resources and expertise to facilitate understanding of patient responsiveness to drug therapies and optimal dosing regimes for a range of therapeutic products.

Essentially, Wyeth envisaged that the work of the collaboration would enable it to best identify the most promising drug candidates in its portfolio as early in development as possible so as to avoid some of the high costs of late-stage failure, which is a problem that plagues the industry as a whole.

The role of the four academic Centres of Excellence was to design and conduct specific TM projects; some of which involved nominated Wyeth compounds. Both NHS Scotland and the Scottish Clinical Research Network were to contribute, in collaboration with the Centres of Excellence, clinical expertise and patient-centred resources relevant to the biomarker studies. The role of the clinical partners was, according to interview respondents from the health service sector, to provide the important link to patients and clinical samples that are considered so crucial to the success of TM. The metaphor of "bench-to-bedside and back again" nicely captures the anticipated relationship between the academic centres and the health service boards.

At the centre of the TMRC was a Central Research Laboratory, located at the University of Dundee. The role of this laboratory was to house technologies and expertise for the analysis of TMRC's clinical research projects carried out at the other academic centres, and also to provide new industry standards for biomarker validation and handling of clinical samples. The laboratory had strong capabilities in transcriptional profiling, proteomics, metabolomics, imaging, analytical biochemistry, biobanking, and bio-informatics/statistics. The Central Research Laboratory comprised

1. A basic research laboratory that provided biomarker discovery, bioinformatics capabilities, assay development, and core service provision to collaborating partners.
2. A clinical laboratory to perform exploratory biomarker studies.
3. A clinical research interface to connect TMRC and the Scottish Clinical Research Network and coordinate activities.

TMRI Ltd was the company established to act as the delivery mechanism for the collaboration and was tasked with two primary functions, according to one interview respondent who was closely involved in its set up. First, TMRI was responsible for distributing the funds from Wyeth and Scottish Enterprise to the collaborating organizations. Second, TMRI had a specific role to exploit outputs from the collaboration, including evaluation and marketing of the Intellectual Property generated from the translational studies. It was also intended that TMRI would broker new translational collaborations with other pharmaceutical and biotechnology firms, which would exploit the same research and clinical infrastructure. The collaboration was set up on a model of shared IP. Although

Wyeth would retain any IP on work directly related to its drug compounds, other drug-related IP would be shared equally, and Scottish Enterprise would retain all IP on any diagnostics and tools developed during the collaboration. This was perhaps where the public sector investor in TMRC saw the ultimate value in the initiative.

Overall coordination and management of the collaboration and its research was conducted by a Steering Committee and Scientific Review Board. Both had representatives from each of the collaborating partners and core funders. The Steering Committee had the important role of determining the broad strategic aims of the collaboration, while the Scientific Review Board was tasked with monitoring and evaluating the individual translational projects.

The scientific program utilized, according to one interview respondent, the following three key approaches; "human exploratory clinical studies" (using disease patients, normal populations, and drug/non drug cohorts); "biomarker research and discovery" (using clinical and preclinical samples to establish efficacy, toxicity, and disease stratification); and "biomarker validation and clinical assay development" (which would link with the development of diagnostic tests).

9.4 Principal Objectives and Contribution to Improving Life Science Innovation

The overarching objective of the TMRC, according to both a number of interview respondents and various press releases at the time of launch, was to develop a world-leading network of clinical and scientific excellence in TM, through the development of core translational projects and the nurturing of new translational activities. However, the collaborating partners also had their own specific objectives.

Interviewees informed me that for Wyeth, the primary aim of TMRC was clearly to accelerate mid-stage drug development so that the risk-profile of compounds could be better identified early in the development pathway. Industry representatives that were interviewed by the author, as well as many of the academic scientists, considered the phase 2 attrition problem faced by all major pharmaceutical companies to be the principal driver of most TM activities. Wyeth appeared to be building its own expectations and visions for TMRC around this core industry challenge. It considered the closer integration of basic and clinical science, with a key emphasis on biomarkers, as a means to achieving this goal of greater phase 2 efficiency and predictability. Wyeth expected to benefit enormously from the access it would gain to external resources and expertise, such as biomarker studies, pharmacogenetics, tissue samples, and clinical trial management. It was hoped that these resources would facilitate the development of its in-house compounds. The collaborative model of TMRC offered a flexible, outsourced organizational structure to facilitate internal R&D, in contrast to the more fundamental experiments in organizational restructuring that have taken place amongst many large pharmaceutical firms over the past couple of decades [1,3,6]; particularity GlaxoSmithKline and the "multi-hub" structure it initiated in 2000 [7,8]. The TMRC model provided for Wyeth an additional strategic option to externally source expertise in parallel to its conventional processes of portfolio and R&D management. Wyeth was exploiting what might be termed a "collaborative network" approach [9], as many large firms have done in response to knowledge and expertise deficits within the life science arena. Its main contribution to the collaboration would be translational capabilities, therapeutic programs, technology leadership, and intellectual property know-how.

The objective of the universities and NHS partners was also to contribute to improvements in the efficiency and effectiveness of biomedical innovation so that new therapeutics and diagnostics could be delivered quickly and safely to patients, but they were also seeking to create critical mass by leveraging greater interaction between the universities and the healthcare system and access new technologies and diagnostic tools for a variety of different purposes. The academic centres would primarily contribute scientific and clinical research expertise and educational mission, while the NHS would provide infrastructure, a patient base, and research programs. In practice, according to many of the academic scientists and clinicians that were interviewed, the universities considered the true value of TMRC in terms of the access to grants and new technologies that participation in the collaboration would unlock. This is perhaps what they prioritized and subsequently built their expectations around. The following quote from an interview with a senior academic scientist nicely illustrates this point.

> "... from an academic perspective what I like is to be able to play with new toys. When I say new toys, obviously I don't mean a new piece of imaging kit or anything like that... they [Wyeth] have a tool, a toy, which is a drug that blocks a receptor or inhibits an enzyme or affects a pathway, which I will never have access to unless I work with them. And then, if I have access to it, that allows me to do and ask innovative questions from a scientific perspective. If that actually in the process then answers their question for their drug TM program, then yes it is worthwhile going taking it to patients, and it's a win–win."

This respondent did, however, proceed to explain that the downside is when the expectations of the different partners do not align. For example, if the academic scientists demonstrate that the drug does not work as intended, this can be invaluable for the pharmaceutical firm, but it does not generate "academic kudos" for the university scientists. This kind of data is not something that can lead to publications in highly rated journals. Nevertheless, a number of the scientists that were interviewed did still consider there to be significant and positive advantages to working on industry projects; particularly in that it adds a new intellectual perspective and can provide new insights. Similarly, interview respondents from the health service side of the collaboration spoke of the broader patient benefits to this kind of large-scale collaborative research and built expectations around the future health benefits for Scotland.

Scottish Enterprise is tasked with improving Scottish economic development and wealth creation. Interviewees suggested that it saw the value of the collaboration primarily in terms of its potential to generate IP for Scotland and further advance the Scottish life science sector to attract further inward investment and create new, globally competitive companies and associated jobs. Similarly, TMRI wanted to exploit the broader benefits of the collaboration and use the resources and infrastructure to leverage further investment from other global pharmaceutical firms.

In terms of outputs, the collaboration was expected to lead to major developments in both diagnostics and therapeutics. It was not, according to the key people involved in the creation of TMRC, seen as a closed drug development collaboration, but a network of highly integrated partnerships combining resources and expertise to improve various aspects of the innovation life cycle. There would be the development of new basic science and clinical methodologies; improvements in the study of biomarkers and processes for validation; as well as standardized processes for ethical approval of clinical trials; and the collection and storage of clinical data. The value was therefore expected to go very much beyond conventional drug development therapeutics.

In both its design and structure, the TMRC was attempting to address a number of specific roadblocks or barriers that continue to undermine health innovation and provide much of the impetus for investment in and development of TM. Two are particularly important. First, for discovery research the collaboration built on and exploited the academic and public research base, including both basic and clinical research. Second, the issue of interoperability and data integration is a particular problem in life science R&D, which was highlighted by an expert in bioinformatics that was interviewed by the author (this respondent had worked both within the pharmaceutical industry and academia). The role of the Central Research Laboratory and the Centres of Excellence to develop new technologies and methods, in partnership with the NHS and clinical networks, was expected to meet this challenge.

The primary strength of TMRC appeared to be its broad integrative strategy for improving the lab–clinic interface to meet some of the challenges of contemporary therapeutic innovation. By combining the resources of a major pharmaceutical company with existing publicly funded institutions and resource infrastructure, the initiative certainly had the potential to become a model of good practice for TM. Wyeth was not simply establishing a new R&D centre or funding a facility or project. Instead, it was buying into an expansive network that would grow and develop over time. Scotland seemed to be a particularly attractive place for this type of collaboration because of its stable and static population; a single healthcare provider, good university and clinical networks, electronic patient health records, established tissue banking facilities, and a world class basic and clinical research base.

The first round of project calls was initiated in May 2006, when more than 80 proposals were submitted. Sixty five programs were supported in the first 2 years and initial reported outputs appeared promising. A number of publications had been published and a strong pipeline of IP opportunities in diagnostics had emerged, including biomarkers of response to neoadjuvant chemotherapy, and novel biomarkers of endometrial dysfunction. However, there were always going to be key challenges facing such a new type of initiative, and the subsequent story of TMRC generates a number of lessons for other public–private collaborations centred on TM.

9.5 Key Challenges Facing the Collaboration and Response to Loss of Follow-on Funding

Although the TMRC had a lot of potential promise in overcoming some of the translational barriers in health innovation, there were always going to be inherent challenges with the potential to usurp the collaborative model. One key weakness of the initiative was that its organizational structure appeared so complex, and some of its objectives rather ambiguous and diverse, that it would always find it difficult to successfully deliver on its early promises. The success of TMRC was always going to be shaped by how well the participating organizations and their research staff would work together on the core research projects and successfully translate the basic science into deliverable products. Furthermore, it was clear from a number of interview accounts that the principal interest of Wyeth was to provide a model for improving its mid-stage R&D efficiency, which was perhaps far less ambitious than some of the other public-sector partners. Indeed, while some key Wyeth representatives spoke at various conferences and workshops very much in terms of cost-savings and efficiency in phase 2 pipelines, the NHS partners and public-sector sponsors spoke far more broadly and speculatively about public health benefit and IP for Scotland when interviewed by the author. While the collaboration was always likely to meet the functional requirements of Wyeth, it was not guaranteed that the broader, and arguably more ambitious goals of the public-sector partners, would ever be fully realized. There were also ever present external factors that threatened to undermine the eventual success of TMRC. Drug development is, by its very nature, subject to much external uncertainty and "Black Swan" events [10]. In particular, market developments and regulatory changes always had the potential to undermine the success of the TMRC.

The TMRC, as indicated earlier, was presented by its proponents as a resounding success in the initial few years of the initiative. Early indications from both the scientists and policymakers directly involved in the collaboration (both those interviewed by the author and others that publicized the initiative in the press) were that the different institutions were linking well together and good scientific work was being conducted. There was also a palpable sense of shared goals and a great deal of institutional buy-in and good will. Nevertheless, there were many challenges in setting up the linkages between the various organizations, and the management of expectations was always going to be difficult, as it perhaps is for all types of public–private partnerships.

Indeed, there are a number of persistent challenges that need to be overcome with any TM approach [11,12], and TMRC was not immune from these. First, complexity of both basic and clinical science, and the institutional and cultural differences between the two, including reward systems, continues to make integration difficult. The academic scientists interviewed often talked about the lack of recognition in academia for work on industry projects that always have the potential to generate negative data on a drug compound that is unpublishable. Others also talked of the difficulty for many academic scientists in working to industry set milestones. The following quote from an R&D director in the NHS is particularly illustrative on this issue.

> Grant-giving bodies, research councils, ok they have their milestones, they ask for their annual reports but they don't actually do an enormous amount if you fail to meet them, until further down the line... And once they've given the money, that's out of their

> system, once they've allocated, even though you don't get it until the next year, and that is not quite the same for the commercial partner. So they are much, much more driven by milestones being met, stringent milestones being met, which is quite hard, some people would find that really hard. And quite demanding, which in an academic environment probably no-one's made allowance for, or sufficient allowance for.

Second, due to the collaborative and interdisciplinary nature of the field, new structural arrangements for academic science, commercial R&D, and regulation are required to facilitate translation, and these aren't always easy to establish and manage. Third, TM (particularly those aspects focused on the genetics of disease) requires greater access to sensitive patient data and tissue samples, where public healthcare systems serve as important gatekeepers and there may be public concern [15,16]. This can conflict with legislation aimed at protecting privacy and intellectual property. Fourth, pharmaceutical companies will always find it difficult to integrate new translational processes with existing R&D pipeline systems, as they try to balance "targeted" and "serendipitous" research and explore the technological challenges of TM and associated areas of research and development. This was a major concern expressed by all the senior R&D managers and scientists in five large global pharmaceutical firms that were interviewed by the author, when exploring the more general impact of life sciences on the organization and management of R&D. Industry had gone through successive waves of experimentation in organizational restructuring and strategy to exploit the new life sciences and sustain product pipelines in the face of technological, scientific, and market uncertainties. Sixth, the interplay between new TM approaches and regulatory systems for new therapies has not so far been sufficiently exploited. There is much greater need and scope for TM and regulatory processes at different stages of drug development to be better aligned so as to facilitate innovation [2], particularly in the emerging field of biomarkers and stratified medicine, which also requires consideration of radically new types of business models and value systems [17].

Finally, the high and often quite divergent expectations for TM, and the broader politics of hype and hope [18], always require careful management. Although in the case of TMRC the goals were not necessarily mutually exclusive, they were never realistically going to be fully aligned. It is therefore important to be sensitive to the importance of reflecting on how different expectations and visions of tangible outcomes can impact on the success of collaborative initiatives in TM. One major issue with regard to TMRC relates to what each of the collaborating partners ultimately expected to get out of their participation. Wyeth appeared to be interested predominantly in exploiting clinical and scientific expertise in the public sector to help progress its compounds along the complex and uncertain drug development pathway. Scottish Enterprise expected valuable IP to be generated for Scotland, although this was never likely to be that significant with a project focused on novel biomarkers, according to one skeptical interview respondent. On the other hand, the expectation that the collaboration would eventually lead to further inward investment in life science and the creation of new jobs and industries was perhaps more realistic. The universities and academics expected access to new technologies and funding, although one must question their commitment to working on "industry focused" projects where there is not always any clear academic benefit, as was illustrated in the interview quote earlier. The NHS expected the collaboration to lead to better treatments for patients. Again, the likelihood of this being a tangible outcome of this particular collaboration was always going to be quite low. Finally, TMRI expected real and tangible benefits in terms of securing further collaborative partners (specifically other multinational pharmaceutical companies) to exploit this growing national resource, but this was always going to prove difficult because, according to one interview respondent, the universities themselves were never under any formal obligation to transact through TMRI and it was never clear what the incentive for doing so would be.

Nevertheless, despite the many challenges, TMRC did at one time exist as a potential exemplar of the broad-based collaborative public–private partnership model that was beginning to emerge in a number of developed nations seeking to spur health innovation. However, TMRC only had guaranteed funding for 5 years (2006–2011), although the business plan was for a 10-year collaboration.

The expectation was that follow-on funding would be made available, and in the early years of the collaboration (when most of the interviews were conducted) many of the people working within TMRC believed this was a long-term collaborative strategy. However, in 2011 it was announced that there would be no further funding. Following the acquisition of the commercial partner Wyeth by Pfizer in October 2009, the future of the TMRC was always going to be uncertain. Mergers and acquisitions in the pharmaceutical sector often lead to divestment of key assets as the acquiring firm imposes post-merger rationalization programs to reduce its cost base and avoid diseconomies of scale [13,14]. Shortly before the first 5-year funding round was due to end in early 2011, the resources within the core research laboratory at Dundee were beginning to be sold as the TMRC announced that it was reviewing its overall structure and business plan. The partners had decided that they no longer wanted to pursue the central lab concept and that research would be now carried out at their own institutions. The TMRC program continued to wind down during 2011 and 2012 as core assets were divested. Despite the fact that follow-on funding was never guaranteed, and there has undoubtedly been some promising scientific outputs from the initial investment, the ending of the initiative was a blow to erstwhile Scottish aspirations to be an international leader in TM activities and a hub for translational collaboration in pharmaceuticals.

9.6 Further Reflections on the Failure of TMRC

The TMRC did not ultimately deliver on all its early promises, but no single reason can fully account for the failure for the initiative and its original vision. A number of related issues contributed to the eventual collapse of the collaboration, and a small number of recent interviews with some key informants have provided some useful insights on this issue.

First, the concept of an integrated, collaborative model involving multiple public and private sector institutions is enticing in theory, but in practice it requires a truly shared vision for the key objectives. It does not appear that this was always the case for TMRC. TMRI should, perhaps, have been better enabled to extract greater value from the resources in terms of transacting with other companies, but the structures didn't seem to be in place to allow this to happen effectively. TMRC always appeared, from the outside, to be a tightly bounded collaboration with few opportunities available for other companies, even if this was not the intention.

Second, translational activities in healthcare require time to fully develop and exploit. A 10–15-year business plan for project development and impact would have been appropriate, but it was always going to be difficult to generate significant scientific results and tradable IP after only 5 years. There was simply not the time to maximize on both the science and economic impact, which is crucial for these kinds of public–private initiatives to be evaluated as successful.

Third, it is important to think critically about the focus on biomarkers, which some people now consider to be at the fringes of TM and unlikely to lead to major breakthroughs or revenue generation in the short term. Identifying and validating biomarkers is certainly important, but to do it right and ensure it translates into improvements in clinical trial design, etc., requires far greater resource infrastructure than that provided by TMRC. One could imagine a large-scale collaboration in the United States involving, for example, the National Institutes of Health (NIH), some of the major academic clinical centres with expertise in phase 3 clinical trials and some large pharma and biotech companies doing something promising in this area. But Scotland did not have the scale and scope to really push forward biomarker and clinical trial development beyond some fairly basic proof of concept work. The question is therefore whether small scale projects such as this can really revolutionize drug development processes and meet the many challenges facing contemporary drug development; particularly the dearth of new therapies making it to the clinic [19].

Fourth, beyond talk of biomarker studies; the aims, objectives, and aspirations of the TMRC partners remained rather vague and ambiguous, which raises serious questions about whether this was ever going to translate into tangible benefits in terms of economic or patient impact. One could argue that a clearer and more achievable range of foci were needed for the collaboration to succeed.

Finally, one cannot underestimate the negative impact that the takeover of Wyeth by Pfizer had on the collaboration, which culminated in Pfizer being unwilling to fund the initiative for a further 5 years. This is always a risk when dealing with a major pharmaceutical company, as strategic priorities can quickly change. However, if the other structural flaws in the initiative had not been present, and TMRI had been able to attract further partners to the central resource, the loss of funding from Pfizer would not necessarily have led to the end of the basic TMRC concept and infrastructure. It could potentially have succeeded in the long-term through a well thought through strategy of organic growth.

9.7 Conclusion: Lessons to be Learned from the TMRC Experience

Within the scientific and clinical communities, as well as the broader policy community, a great deal of faith is continuing to be placed in the success of new types of translational models for health innovation. It is clear that the conventional approach to drug development is unsustainable as no one firm has the range of technologies, knowledge, expertise, and complementary assets to develop therapies entirely in-house. In the life sciences particularly, firms must collaborate with other organizations, as well as academic centres and clinical networks to bridge the gap between basic and clinical science and bring new products to market. TM by its very nature demands models like TMRC; in theory if not necessarily in practice.

Although TMRC ultimately ended in failure, there were some positive outcomes. TMRC did help to initiate a process to transform some of the governance structures for health research in Scotland; for example, streamlining ethical approvals for research and clinical trials; and it did provide a new level of research excellence and standardization for the development of biomarker studies. The individual projects that were funded also generated new knowledge and technologies and perhaps some valuable IP that may still be exploited in the future. However, one might argue that much of this could have been achieved through other means. The collaboration essentially promised more than it could realistically deliver and this case study provides a number of important lessons for TM and the collaborative structures needed to drive it forward.

First, public sector economic development agencies need to think carefully about the extent to which they fund risky, early stage translational research initiatives, as opposed to supporting small companies and broader industrial development.

Second, there is an issue about the extent to which TM requires new technologies and ideas in basic translational science, including early biomarker work, rather than better translational processes for commercializing technologies that are already available and close to market.

Third, the scale, scope, and focus of any collaborative project must be agreed early in the process by all the partners and the broad strategic vision must be shared. Otherwise, it is very difficult to ensure these initiatives gain traction and provide long-term value in terms of both health benefit and economic impact.

Finally, a TM initiative that has good institutional buy-in, shared aims and objectives; excellent science and sound governance structures should not be liable to collapse if one key source of funding abruptly ends. Broad-based, public–private initiatives aimed at facilitating translation of basic science into clinically effective products need time to grow and deliver on the promises and expectations they create. They are unlikely to succeed when under intense pressure to deliver significant results in the short term, especially when there are many diverse and often misaligned hopes, expectations, and research and development cultures, which this case study has highlighted.

References

1. Mittra, J. (2008). Impact of the life sciences on organisation and management of R&D in large pharmaceutical firms, *International Journal of Biotechnology*, **10** (5), pp. 416–440.

2. Mittra, J., Tait, J., and. Wield, D. (2011). From maturity to high value-added innovation: lessons from the pharmaceutical and agro-biotechnology industries, *Trends in Biotechnology*, **29** (3), pp. 105–109.
3. Mittra, J. (2007). Life science innovation and the re-structuring of the pharmaceutical sector: mergers, acquisitions and strategic alliances, *Technology Analysis and Strategic Management*, **19** (3), pp. 279–301.
4. Gambardella, A., *et al.* (2000). *Global Competitiveness in Pharmaceuticals: A European Perspective*, Report Prepared for the Directorate General Enterprise of the European Commission, November 2000.
5. Scottish Enterprise (2005). *Scottish Life Sciences Strategy: Achieving Critical Mass*, Scottish Enterprise Report, February 15 2005 http://www.scotland.gov.uk/Resource/Doc/37428/0009610.pdf (accessed July, 2011).
6. Cockburn, I.M. (2004). The changing structure of the pharmaceutical industry, *Health Affairs*, **23** (1), pp. 10–22.
7. Huckman, R., and Strick, E. (2005). GlaxoSmithKline: reorganizing drug discovery (A), *Harvard Business School Case Study*, 9-605-074, May 2005.
8. Criscuolo, P. and Narula, R. (2007). Using multi-hub structures for international R&D: Organisational inertia and the challenges of implementation, *Managerial International Review*, **5**, October 2007.
9. Chiesa, V. and Toletti, G. (2004). Network of collaborations for innovation: the case of biotechnology, *Technology Analysis and Strategic Management*, **16** (1), pp. 73–96.
10. Tait, J. (2009) *The Pharmaceutical Industry: Bio-engineering a "Black Swan," Britain in 2009*. ESRC Publication, p 84.
11. Pober, J., Neuhauser, C., and Pober, J. (2001). Obstacles facing translational research in academic medical centers. *The Federation of American Societies for Experimental Biology Journal*, **15**, pp. 2303–2313.
12. Horig, H. Marincola, E., and Marincola, F. (2005). Obstacles and opportunities in translational research. *Nature Medicine*, **11** (7), pp. 705–708.
13. Henderson, R. and Cockburn, I. (1997). *Firm Size and Research Productivity in Drug Discovery*, 1997 (available at http://www.mit.edu/afs/athena/course/15/15.141/readings/insee97.pdf (accessed July 2011).
14. Allen, P., Ramlogan, R., and Randles, S. (2002). Complex systems and the merger process, *Technology Analysis and Strategic Management*, **14** (3), pp. 315–329.

15. Smith, B., *et al.* (2006). Generation Scotland: The Scottish Family Health Study: A new resource for researching genes and heritability, *BMC Medical Genetics*, 7 (74), doi:10.1186/1471-2350-7-74.
16. Haddow, G., *et al.* (2011). Can the governance of a population genetic data bank effect recruitment? Evidence from the public consultation of Generation Scotland, *Public Understanding of Science*, **20** (1), pp. 117–129.
17. Mittra, J. and Tait, J. (2012). Analysing stratified medicine business models and value systems: innovation-regulation interactions, *New Biotechnology*, (in press, http://dx.doi.org/10.1016/j.nbt.2012.03.003).
18. Borup, M., *et al.* (2006). The sociology of expectations in science and technology, *Technology Analysis and Strategic Management*, **18** (3,4), pp. 285–298.
19. Anon (2011). Where will new drugs come from?, *The Lancet*, 377, January 8, 2011.

Chapter 10

The Role of the Product Development Partnership as a Translational Mechanism for Delivering Health Solutions in Low-Resource Settings[†]

Julius Mugwagwa,[*] Rebecca Hanlin, Joanna Chataway, and Lois Muraguri

Innogen Centre, Development Policy and Practice, Faculty of Maths, Computing and Technology, The Open University, Walton Hall, Milton Keynes, MK7 6AA, UK

*j.t.mugwagwa@open.ac.uk

10.1 Introduction

In this chapter we describe and discuss the International AIDS Vaccine Initiative (IAVI) as a case study for understanding the emerging role of health product development partnerships (PDPs) in providing new solutions to health problems in low-resource settings. Based on a broader analysis of the emergence and impact of global health partnerships, this chapter highlights the need

[†]This chapter is adapted from a paper by the same authors, Global Health Social Technologies: Reflections on evolving theories and landscapes, *Research Policy*, 39, pp. 1277–1288.

Translational Medicine: The Future of Therapy
Edited by James Mittra and Christopher-Paul Milne

ISBN 978-981-4316-99-6 (Hardback), 978-981-4364-84-3 (eBook)
www.panstanford.com

for multidisciplinary and multi-institutional approaches, which are exemplified by IAVI and similar PDPs, and considers the extent to which these translational approaches are leading the way in terms of developing new vaccines for HIV/AIDS and other neglected diseases. The contextual historical, organizational, and scientific issues surrounding these efforts are presented and discussed in this chapter, leading to our conclusion that PDPs such as the IAVI are playing increasingly crucial roles in translational medicine (TM) within developing countries.

Delivering effective and sustainable health care rests on the ability to successfully transform laboratory findings into new ways of diagnosing and treating patients, and supporting programs and infrastructure to improve the health of populations worldwide. This process, which we broadly define as TM, encapsulates, amongst other things, social, technological, ethical, regulatory, and geographical boundaries and challenges that need to be addressed.

Health delivery remains an onerous challenge in both developed and developing countries, but in developing countries there are additional resource challenges that have led to systemic weakness in health delivery programs. In these countries, health policy must start with strengthening the health care system infrastructure so that healthcare solutions can be efficiently implemented. However, strengthening the health care system in low-resource settings is a daunting challenge. Furthermore, the nature of the challenges can be highly variable between countries, and the definition of what even constitutes a 'health system' in one setting may be very different from what it is in another. Developing universal solutions to these health care challenges is problematic, but on the other hand, bespoke solutions (health technologies included) are expensive and time consuming. Ultimately, if sustainable health systems that address the needs of all people requiring health care are to emerge, they must be compatible with local social and clinical contingencies and recognize the importance of existing institutional and policy norms and arrangements for engaging recipient communities.

Our focus in this chapter is IAVI, a health product development partnership that we have been working with to explore how public–

Box 10.1 Product development partnerships defined.

> Many PDPs were established in the mid-1990s to help address the 10/90 gap — that only 10% of health research funding was targeted towards diseases that accounted for 90% of the global disease burden (GFHR, 2004). While each PDP operates differently depending on the disease area(s) of focus, they typically employ a portfolio approach to R&D to accelerate product development by pursuing multiple strategies for the same disease area. They also work in close partnership with academia, large pharmaceutical companies, the biotechnology industry, and governments in developing countries. Although PDPs typically use private industry approaches to portfolio management, they focus on disease areas that lack viable commercial markets. PDPs with products in advanced stages of development have also focused additional efforts on ensuring equitable access and uptake of new products they have helped develop. (*Source:* IAVI Insight Policy Brief, Sept 2010)

private partnerships might work as vehicles for exploiting TM and policy development in a developing world context. Box 10.1 provides a short definition of a PDP. This initiative is one of many that are attempting to harness technological developments in the developed world to address neglected diseases affecting the world's poorest populations. These different initiatives employ novel forms of technology development and institutional arrangements aimed at delivering solutions to the affected populations, including knowledge brokerage and integration [1]. Through the IAVI case study we hope to broaden understanding of the complexity and unique challenges of TM and health care delivery in developing countries, explore the justification for particular approaches to the development and delivery of new therapies, and begin to think through how some of the approaches might be optimized and made to work in the context of continuing shifts in science, technology, and innovation practices and priorities; and the more recent drop in funding and investment options due to the global financial crisis.

10.2 Background and Context

Developing countries, particularly those in Africa, suffer from a significant disease burden. The World Health Organization (WHO) estimates that malaria, which disproportionately affects children and those living in Africa, kills 1.2 million people a year and that nearly 3.2 billion people a year are affected by a single bout of malaria. Nearly 40 million people throughout the world are infected with HIV/AIDS, and 65% of all new infections occur in Africa. A number of lesser-known diseases, such as human African Trypanosomiasis, Chagas disease, and Leishmaniasis, also add significantly to the disease burden in Africa. Categorized as 'neglected diseases', the latter attract much less funding and attention than HIV/AIDS and malaria, yet they still have a dire impact on many African populations [2].

Scientific and technological innovation in the area of health can go some way towards reducing Africa's disease burden (see Box 10.2). One example has been the development of Highly Active Anti-Retroviral Therapy (HAART), which has increased the survival rates of those with HIV/AIDS. Although it does not cure the disease, drug treatment of HIV does significantly increase life expectancy and is seen as being partly responsible for reduction in the international AIDS mortality rate. Advances in water purification technology have also had a significant impact on public health by enabling evermore people access to safe drinking water. More high-tech innovations in genomics and molecular biology are also driving new developments in drug, vaccine, and diagnostics.

Box 10.2 Africa's health care challenge — an overview.

- High disease burden, including rapid spread and persistence of killer diseases, e.g. HIV/AIDS, tuberculosis, and malaria
- Deteriorating health infrastructure (for training and health delivery services)
- Low and declining investments in health research
- Loss of health personnel (due to diseases and through 'brain drain')
- Poor regulation of the health care sector

However, improving public health is a hugely complex and challenging process. It relies, in part, on products that work reaching the people who need them most. In addition to the significant scientific challenges involved in tackling disease, there must be a market demand to fund product development. Once a product is finally developed, an effective health system with appropriate infrastructure and skilled staff are needed to successfully deliver the therapy. Crucially, these products must be affordable to what are some of the world's poorest people. In their endeavour to bridge technology and product gaps for neglected diseases and other health challenges in the global south, PDPs are playing a critical role in TM.

10.3 Innovating for Health and the Growth of PDPS

A key notion underpinning TM is that some of the traditional practices of drug development and delivery need to be changed or adapted if therapeutic innovations are to bring about effective health solutions to the problems faced by developing countries. An examination of the history and growth of PDPs confirms that significant changes have indeed occurred regarding the practice of R&D and funding of new technologies and products for neglected diseases over the past three decades. Generally, health R&D in the post-war period was characterized by a division of labor where basic research was conducted by universities and other public research institutions, while the private sector focused on applied research. The typical multinational pharmaceutical company engaged in more applied R&D as well as manufacturing the drugs it produced [3].

The 1970s witnessed the first attempts at collaboration between the public and private sectors in health R&D. Attempts by the private sector to collaborate with the public sector (particularly universities) created early opportunities for addressing the basic-applied and public–private dichotomies. Prior to the late 1970s, it was argued that there was little reason to believe that such collaborative practices were 'substantially associated with important productivity gains for firms' [4]. However, in the following decades greater capacity in biology and biochemistry within public institutions was complemented by a move from random screening towards a more science-oriented "rational" drug design within commercial pharmaceutical companies.

> Firms who adopted this approach shifted their research activities to rely increasingly on theories about the biological basis of disease. In order to access such findings, science-oriented firms began to allow (and even encourage) their researchers to interact more closely with the scientific community external to the firm, including publishing in the public scientific literature. [4]

The shift from random screening to "drug discovery by design" depended on the ability of commercial firms to source and exploit publicly generated knowledge [4, 5]. An assessment of 21 of the most influential therapeutic drugs between 1965 and 1992 by Cockburn and Henderson [6] found that public sector input was essential to private sector drug discovery and development. This suggests that the ability to access and interact with the public sector was an important determinant of private sector productivity in downstream research.

Success in applied research became more dependent on an understanding of basic research [7]. Fundamental advances in the life sciences in the 1980s led to a widening of the health R&D 'participatory space' with the rise of the specialist private sector biotechnology companies. This changed the dynamics of health R&D.

> ... the revolution in biomedical science and genetics has posed greater threats to the mainstream pharmaceutical industry because of its potential to make some of the key competences that the industry has irrelevant. [7]

Health R&D in the 1990s was characterized by the rise of biotech firms that acted as upstream suppliers of technology to pharmaceutical companies, and a substantial growth in subcontracting by major pharmaceutical companies at various stages of the R&D process [7]. The rise of the biotech companies could be seen as a response to the technological opportunities created by new scientific knowledge. In response to the new challenges presented by the biotech companies, the pharmaceutical firms sought to acquire the companies, to develop their own in-house biotech capacity or to build strategic alliances [8], including subcontracting work to the biotech firms.

Two observations can be made about the evolution of health R&D up to the late 1990s. First, developments from the 1970s show not only how new entrants gained access to the health R&D field, but also how the actors at any given time related to each other. Thus the strict dichotomy of roles and division of labor between public sector basic research and private sector applied research in the post-war period was followed by closer collaboration between the two sectors from the 1970s, and then a new division of labor emerged between biotech firms and pharmaceutical companies in the 1980s and 1990s.

Second, there has been a gradual widening of the 'participatory space' that has allowed new entrants into the field. This may have been sparked by advances in science and technology, as was the case in the biotech firms, but also by the growing demand for new institutions to take on some of the work that had hitherto been undertaken by the large pharmaceutical companies. Companies were subcontracted by big pharma as there was growing recognition that the current actors in health R&D could not, in isolation, meet broader health goals; hence the emergence of PDPs.

The blurring of the boundary between the private and the public, as well as between research and development, increasingly led to new PDPs involving the public and private sector. PDPs are in themselves new translational institutions that occupy part of the broadening 'participatory space' in health R&D. They constitute an innovative mechanism through which the public and private sectors can relate to each other and work towards the achievement of a specified goal. They may be seen as an organizational experiment to better bridge the gap between established institutional actors and their diverse R&D foci.

The notion that PDPs could significantly improve health innovation for neglected diseases gained currency in the late 1990s with the establishment of IAVI. Prior to the official launch of IAVI, various meetings were arranged to identify and evaluate the barriers to HIV/AIDS vaccine development, which provided the impetus for the establishment of a radically different approach. IAVI emerged from growing concern that little progress had been made towards the development of a vaccine; especially in a developing country context [9].

The rationalizations and principal motives underpinning IAVI, particularly the lack of any existing mechanisms to deliver these specific healthcare solutions, also demonstrate the need and impetus for using the PDP approach in other related contexts.

> Those who participated in the founding of IAVI believed that the NIH was focused almost exclusively on basic science and would not expeditiously develop vaccines for HIV/AIDS, especially vaccines that met the needs of the developing world. Nor did they envisage other national science establishments that would develop a vaccine in the near term. In addition, they believed that the private sector did not see a market for such vaccines. They were also certain that even if such a vaccine were developed by the private sector that it would be unaffordable for those who needed it most. [10]

PDPs are part of a broader global movement towards a collaboration and partnership strategy for healthcare research and development. PDPs have now been joined by a variety of other types of global health partnerships that bring together public and private sector partners with different sets of functions and objectives [11]. One global health partnership, the Global Alliance for Vaccines and Immunisation (GAVI), was established in 2000 in response to the challenges presented by immunization. Immunization levels were dropping in many countries and some preventable diseases were re-emerging. It hoped to revive the Expanded Programme on Immunization, which had been inspired by the success of the smallpox eradication programme in the 1970s. GAVI's business plan is premised on market intervention; the idea being that since the poor in developing countries cannot pay GAVI should provide the finance. As the Executive Secretary of GAVI has stated

> GAVI was formed in 2000 for those poor countries — for the poorest of the poor — the 70-odd countries with a gross national income of under US$ 1000. They are not the traditional view

> of a promising market. Especially not for any product which requires enormous upfront investment in research development and testing. What happens when you change perspective — when you view the disease burden of the developing world as the market and the people of that world as worthy of investment? What happens when you consolidate all those populations into one giant market and relocate your view of purchasing power — from them, to GAVI? It means that you gain market shaping capability. It means you can create new dynamics of supply and demand that get the newest vaccines to the countries that need them most. Much, much sooner... prices decline as the volume of demand, consolidated through GAVI, makes production investment worthwhile for manufacturers. More manufacturers enter the market with better demand forecasts, and a beneficial cycle begins. [12] (emphasis in original).

The argument for global health partnerships, and especially PDPs, is in part informed by the rationale of missing incentives and market failure arguments, although this does not account for the whole picture. The creation of PDPs goes beyond the market failure argument, because these new entities constitute much more than tools for incentivizing and attracting private sector input; they bring together public and private organizations and individuals in new forms of social interaction. We consider PDPs to be social experiments [13]; that is, they are products of organizational and institutional reforms aimed at dealing with the unique problems and technology and health needs of the poor. In this sense, they are very good examples of TM; exploiting novel institutional mechanisms and capacity-building approaches to bridge some of the gaps in health research and delivery in low resource settings. PDPs provide multi-actor integrated solutions required by the ever broader scope and complexity of today's health problems [14]. Furthermore, they help build a contained collective capacity to respond 'to turbulent conditions as creative solutions are needed that exceed the limited perspectives of each individual partner' [15].

The synergy concept is underpinned by the assumption that partnership arrangements can achieve more than the individual agents involved could independently. This is particularly so in health PDPs. Advocating for 'push' and 'pull' mechanisms to address the production of vaccines for the poor, Smith points out:

> The public sector alone cannot solve the problem because almost all new vaccines and drugs come from private companies. Yet private companies cannot solve the problem alone because their obligations to their shareholders mean seeking the highest returns, which tend to come from developing products for the rich world. [16]

By the end of 2004, global health partnerships, including PDPs, were responsible for nearly 75% of neglected disease drug development projects [17]; indicating that they have provided the impetus for renewed activity in research on drugs for neglected diseases.

10.4 The Funding Context

At the same time that PDPs have been gaining in popularity, there have been significant changes in the funding regime for new technologies and products for neglected diseases. Increased investment from both the private sector and various foundations and other not-for-profit organizations has occurred in parallel with the rise of PDPs. Foundations have been integral to the development of many PDPs. For example, early meetings that led to the creation of IAVI were convened by the Rockefeller Foundation, which also provided the initial funding. IAVI subsequently received substantial funding from the Bill and Melinda Gates Foundation (BMGF). Without this early support from the BMGF, it is unlikely that IAVI would have established itself as the pre-eminent force that not only made a significant contribution to raising awareness of the need for and possibility of developing an AIDS vaccine [10], but also became a model of good practice for the establishment of other PDPs. IAVI did not rely entirely on the early financial support of the Gates Foundation, but was proactive and successful in bringing in money from other donors such as the Foundation of National Institutes of Health, and development agencies such as the UK's Department for International Development (DfID). One senior manager in a development agency has described PDPs as 'low hanging fruit' [13]; meaning they are a relatively easy and effective way for development agencies and donors to spend money. PDPs were set up with the credibility of being backed by major institutions. Also, because they tended to be professionally organized and managed, this made it easier for donor agencies to justify their often substantial investments.

Similarly, PATH's Malaria Vaccine Initiative (MVI) was established in 1999 through an initial grant by the BMGF, which continues to be its main source of funding although MVI also receives support from USAID and ExxonMobil. Early partners in the exploratory discussions leading to the launch of Medicines for Malaria Venture (MMV) included the Rockefeller Foundation and the International Federation of Pharmaceutical Manufacturers Association. These, along with ExxonMobil, the Global Forum for Health Research and other traditional donors provide financial support for MMV. In 1999, the GAVI Alliance received a start up grant of US$750m from the BMGF.

These examples illustrate the diversification in global financing of health R&D away from the traditional development assistance donors. The recent establishment of mechanisms such as the International Finance Facility for Immunisation (IFFIm), which borrows on capital markets against donor countries' pledges to raise funds through issuing bonds, illustrates the new impetus and energy around financing neglected diseases. By 2007, funds collected from IFFIm represented 29% of the total funds, close to the BMGF's 30% [18].

According to the estimates provided by the Global Forum for Health Research, the private for-profit sector investment globally in health R&D accounted for 51% of the total global investments in 2005. Governments accounted for 41% of overall funds. Although accounting for only 8% of the total global investment in health R&D, the private not-for-profit sector, which includes foundations, recorded the largest increase in investment between 1998 and 2005. For low- and middle-income countries, the private not-for-profit sector accounted for 10% of the funds invested in health

R&D in 2005 [3]. Foundations and other private not-for-profit actors therefore remain key global partners in global health R&D and TM.

10.5 PDPS as Social and Organizational Experiments in TM

A lot has been achieved in global health R&D since the introduction of PDPs and the unprecedented generosity of non-traditional donors such as foundations and philanthropic organizations. Social and organizational experiments have yielded innovative institutions and increased investment in global health, which has subsequently resulted in the 'fattest pipeline of new technological innovation for diseases primarily affecting resource-poor environments that the world has ever seen' [19]. Perhaps as importantly, and certainly as a consequence of intentional effort on the part of PDPs, there is a political momentum to address major infectious neglected diseases in new nexuses of social cooperation. However, in many cases the products of this novel combination of physical and social technologies are not being delivered quickly enough to those most in need. The reason for this is what we consider a major translational gap; that is weak or non-existent healthcare infrastructure and basic systems in low resource settings, which are the main targets for research in neglected diseases. Elias summarizes the problem as follows:

> Recent investments in new technology development have not yet been matched by similar efforts to strengthen health systems in resource-poor settings. The danger is that new innovations will not move smoothly into widespread use, even in places where they are desperately needed, because of weaknesses in health systems… Failure to bring new products into use could also become a disincentive for the creative partnerships that drive the development of innovations for the poor. [19]

This potential problem has already been picked up by some global health partnerships. One of the four goals of the GAVI Alliance is to 'contribute to strengthening the capacity of the health system to deliver immunisation and other health services in a sustainable manner'. To this end, the GAVI Alliance has committed US$800m over a 5-year period dedicated to strengthening health systems. Although IAVI does not have health systems strengthening as an explicit goal in the way that the GAVI Alliance does, its work on capacity building in conducting clinical trials can be seen as contributing to the need for stronger and better resourced health delivery systems with appropriately skilled staff. We expect to see this agenda explicitly taken on board by some partnerships, at least as PDPs evolve and progress. We return to this key issue later in the chapter.

10.6 Understanding the Integrator and Broker Framework

As the above analysis makes clear, there is considerable turbulence and uncertainty in the organization of efforts to produce and distribute vaccines and new drugs for neglected diseases in low resource settings. PDPs have emerged to fill a vacuum in which traditional public and private organizations alone were either unwilling or unable to operate successfully in this context. In this section, we explore in more detail the institutional form that PDPs represent and suggest an 'integrator and broker' framework as a useful heuristic device for understanding their activities. Innovation studies tend to view innovation (meaning the successful commercialization or distribution of a new product) as the outcome of processes of integration between research and development (R&D), manufacturing, and marketing and distribution activities. Although these processes involve many diverse organizations and institutions, one can often detect a pattern of control. Orsenigo *et al.* address this with reference to pharmaceuticals:

> If one considers drugs for instance, despite the growing trend towards outsourcing and inter-organisational collaborations, large pharmaceutical companies play a central role in coordinating the different elements of the innovation process, including managing

> increasingly demanding regulatory approval processes across a widening spectrum of actors. [1]

The authors note that there is a convincing body of literature showing that in a variety of science and engineering industries a relatively large company gradually establishes itself as a 'hub' co-ordinating the activities of a widely distributed body of innovators. They become 'integrators'. Orsenigo explains:

> The reasons for the prevalence of this configuration are various, and may reflect a long standing balance of power among industry participants rooted in history or tradition. However, this configuration has also been shown to be particularly suitable to enable problem solving in a context in which the underlying knowledge bases (e.g. scientific disciplines) are rapidly evolving and differentiating. [1]

'Hubs' or integrators emerge to organize disparate actors around the complex feedback loops of trial and error requiring highly specialized knowledge. It is usually the case that as the integrator establishes itself it becomes less open to a broad spectrum of ideas and more committed to a single course of action. Orsenigo *et al.* note that since 1945 the organization of vaccine production has differed from that of other sectors. They point out that two 'regulatories' can be observed in the organization of vaccine innovation since 1945. 'The first is that the "invention" element of the innovation process (discovery) typically takes place in public sector institutions (particularly universities). The second is that at a certain point along the development process, there is a hand over to industry. In very few instances is it possible to identify a single institution, whether public or private, acting as the hub across the whole process' [1].

Orsenigo *et al.* suggest that PDPs might be evolving to take on that role in different disease areas. However, they note that the way forward is far from certain and in looking at the PDPs' role more holistically, it becomes clear that PDPs are not only innovators and integrators but also undertake the role of 'broker'. Brokering is seen here as bringing together actors around a set of objectives, sharing information, and facilitating cooperation, with the necessary feedback loops that are a critical component of translational research. It is a role performed by agencies and organizations involved in development work, which is essential for carrying out the work of technology and drug development in developing country contexts. The knowledge brokerage role of PDPs can be observed in their advocacy activities at national and international levels, in their policy work, and their role in bringing together different actors and required expertise for the conduct of clinical trials. PDPs also play a key role in generating 'political demand' for health products and treatments where economic demand is lacking. Brokerage activities require an active and committed presence in developing countries. It is for this reason that bilateral donors such as DfID have been willing to generously fund these activities.

So far we have suggested that PDPs represent a new vehicle for TM R&D in developing countries, trying to successfully combine and coordinate science, technology, innovation, and socio-economic development activities in the fight against neglected diseases. We have looked at PDPs as having both 'integrator and broker' characteristics. However, it is still unclear in which direction PDPs will continue to evolve. In their innovation activities, they are being pulled in two distinct directions. On the one hand they will act as broad-based brokers, but on the other hand they tend towards becoming 'integrator hubs'. What is interesting is that not all PDPs are evolving in the same direction. In the following section, we trace the evolution of IAVI and reveal how it has strengthened its role as a key actor in TM.

10.7 The Changing Global Health Landscape

IAVI, like many other institutional actors, exists in a rapidly changing global health landscape with multiple challenges. First, there is a recurring emphasis on strengthening health systems and the need to build up primary health care in developing countries. This creates potential problems for PDPs as they must increasingly compete for continued funding with those initiatives to better distribute existing products that can have an immediate impact on disease reduction and can be used to strengthen health service provision.

Second, the world financial crisis is putting increased pressure on PDPs' resources, while there is increasing disillusionment amongst some donors with regard to the slow scientific progress being made by PDPs in some key areas. These pressures are leading to increased competition between PDPs and other global health partnerships. Third, as PDPs respond to the slow scientific progress and begin to shift some of their activities more upstream towards applied and basic science, they must continually demonstrate that they remain active and retain links on the ground in developing countries to sustain their position as bridges between innovation and development activities. Finally, even where PDPs have had success in developing new drugs and medicines, this can bring new challenges relating to standardization, regulation, manufacturing, and delivery, which rely heavily on adequate and functioning infrastructure and expertise being in place. Therefore PDPs, as new social technologies or 'organizational mixes', will need to adapt as they interact with the broader institutional environment and its fluctuating resource capacities and competencies [3].

IAVI was initiated in 1996 as a not-for-profit organization based in New York City. On the one hand it acts as a type of 'virtual pharmaceutical company', but it also conducts activities very similar to an international development agency. It is this combination of activities and institutional cultures that enables IAVI to act as both an integrator of scientific knowledge and also a knowledge broker, particularly around issues of advocacy and HIV vaccine preparedness communications within developing countries.

Following initial work as an advocacy organization — mainly raising awareness of the need for funding of AIDS vaccine research, IAVI then focused on becoming actively involved in AIDS vaccine research. This started as a brokering role, in that IAVI tried to provide an organizational entity around which others within the AIDS vaccine community could coalesce. For example, since 1998 IAVI has published a scientific blueprint document that highlights the key areas of research being undertaken, reports on candidate vaccines being tested, and suggests where scientific research should move in the future. To illustrate, on the website page for the 2008 Blueprint, entitled '*A Challenge to the Field, A Roadmap for Progress*, IAVI writes that the Blueprint:

> aims to set the record straight about the current state of AIDS vaccine research and development and offers a series of interim targets to bring the field closer to *the ultimate goal — a safe, effective and accessible AIDS vaccine*. [20]

IAVI has also set up a venture capitalist-type fund, called the Innovation Fund, which since 2007 has provided small amounts of capital to biotechnology companies in order to stimulate research in neglected or marginal areas that IAVI feels are important areas to pursue but aren't being supported by other organizations.

> IAVI's Innovation Fund, the most recent addition to its state-of-the-art program, aims to encourage experimentation on pioneering ideas in ways that other funding sources available today have not, infusing AIDS vaccine science with novel approaches. Targeted primarily to small- and medium-sized biotech companies, the Fund is intended to attract fresh ideas from beyond the mainstream HIV field in an effort to accelerate the development of a preventive AIDS vaccine... Projects considered for IAVI's Innovation Fund must, first and foremost, have the potential to impact ongoing AIDS vaccine research, if successful. Second, they must have the ability to generate preliminary data demonstrating feasibility within the funding period of 12–18 months. Finally, priority will be given to projects that are not currently funded and would not typically be eligible for funding through existing channels for AIDS vaccine development. [21]

Increasingly, IAVI has become more of a knowledge integrator, moving from promoting science done by others to building its own laboratories within which to conduct basic and applied research. This appears at odds with the strategy adopted by many large pharmaceutical firms, which in recent years have embarked on a strategy of buying in or contracting out a lot of basic research; particularly by engaging in partnerships with smaller biotechnology firms [3]. One of the most illustrative examples of how IAVI has moved towards being a scientific integrator is in the scientific area of neutralizing antibodies.

In 2002 IAVI established the Neutralizing Antibody Consortium. The NAC, as it is known, was founded to consolidate research around this neglected area of vaccine science and development. Similar to its more recent Innovation Fund, through the NAC IAVI has acted as a form of venture capitalist; providing funds for researchers to work in this area but also providing a shared means of communication for IAVI funded researchers. The NAC brings together all the major researchers in this area, including the US National Institutes of Health (NIH), which is by far the largest funder of HIV/AIDS vaccine research globally.

When NAC began, it was an example of IAVI simply brokering knowledge by using its position to acquire new knowledge and bring together others who had not considered it. However, IAVI began to introduce an integrator focus by actively coordinating the various actors. Add to this its broader desire to create an AIDS vaccine consortium and operate in-house laboratories for applied research and the argument that IAVI is operating increasingly as a knowledge integrator becomes ever more convincing. The idea of a large vaccine consortium was based not on the notion that IAVI would manage this entity in-house, but that it would promote an industrial project management effort linking leading companies, laboratories, and other research organizations from around the world. The consortium would work to solve all the scientific challenges facing AIDS vaccine research and work together to quickly develop the required solutions.

The laboratories, on the other hand, were envisaged to be IAVI's own in-house laboratories. They demonstrate, we argue, an almost complete re-visioning of IAVI from scientific knowledge broker to integrator. The lab became operational in 2007 in leased lab space within a new bioscience centre at Brooklyn Army Terminal. It took a further year to get the lab operational and the AIDS Vaccine Design and Development Laboratory officially opened. The lab has been described by IAVI as the "only facility in the world to be dedicated exclusively to the design and development of an AIDS vaccine" [22]. The lab is affiliated to the State University of New York and is expected to work in close collaboration with others (such as the NAC), to close the translational research gap created by disincentives within the commercial sector to take forward basic research through to clinical development in areas such as HIV/AIDS. As outlined in the press release for the opening of the lab:

> The lab's scientists, with external partners, will explore innovative ideas from academia, basic research and beyond, using the tried and true methods of industry to speed the development of a public good: an AIDS vaccine for use throughout the world. [22]

These examples highlight how IAVI has successfully strengthened its in-house capabilities and turned the idea of being a public–private incubator of new vaccine candidates into a reality.

10.8 IAVI in Developing Countries

While IAVI is taking on the characteristics of a knowledge integrator in the area of AIDS vaccine research, this is not the case in terms of its work in developing countries and in the global health arena around advocacy and communications for AIDS vaccine work. Here, IAVI still exhibits itself as a knowledge broker, shaping the agenda and providing voice and capabilities for new or previously unheard actors and institutions. This role is very much based on IAVI's understanding of the need to work in collaboration with developing countries. IAVI learned early on through problems with its initial clinical trials in Kenya and India that it needed to be seen as both an inclusive and committed partner, rather than an external US-based company imposing technological fixes from afar. IAVI therefore places much emphasis on allowing others to take the lead. It is a participant, rather than the central node, in a network made up of government and non-governmental agencies including research organizations, local communities, and industry, among others. This is how IAVI conducts much of its advocacy work both in developing countries, in preparation for clinical trials, and at an international level in discussions around the AIDS vaccine and neglected disease policy agendas. In both cases the emphasis is on facilitating the activities of other nodes, be it a local government regulatory authority in developing best practice clinical trial guidelines, or international debates around Advance Market Commitments.

A good example of this is IAVI's work in the area of HIV vaccine literacy. IAVI understands the need to support an increasingly internationally held view that in order for clinical trials to take place effectively, and for adequate demand for a potential vaccine to be created, communities affected by HIV/AIDS need to be aware of both what a vaccine is and can do and the dangers of HIV/AIDS as a disease. Thus, IAVI has worked to develop, in collaboration with its partners around the world, what are known as 'core materials'. This is an information pack, which becomes the backbone of all IAVI-related HIV vaccine literacy work. The information pack outlines information on HIV/AIDS (its transmission, prevention, and treatment) as well as current AIDS vaccine research strategies and details of how a trial of a vaccine works in practice. Crucially, IAVI allows practitioners on the ground to use and modify these materials as needed. This recognition and respect given to local context and contingency is a key requirement for success in overcoming translational health gaps in developing countries.

These knowledge and literacy activities mean IAVI is taking on responsibilities similar to an international development agency with a focus on public health. Similarly, IAVI increasingly has to consider questions of HIV prevention and treatment programs in its clinical trial operations. In these situations IAVI also works to bring together often previously disconnected organizations so that discussions can take place about how best to ensure or reinvigorate healthcare provision or HIV prevention and treatment programs.

10.9 Discussion and Conclusions

IAVI presents itself as having both knowledge integrator and knowledge broker qualities, and sees no problem in these evolving over time as the organization and its members change and adapt to new challenges and opportunities. The hybrid nature of IAVI is the result of both history and cultural evolution within the organization and the way in which these interrelate. The resulting 'institutional logics' [23] are the result of the wider environmental pressures which are then affected by practical activity (in this case the working together of individuals from different backgrounds on tasks that have differing foci of either science or development) and then reproduced and reformulated through that activity [24].

The current nature of IAVI can be seen partly as a consequence of its historical development, because the evolution of IAVI is bound up in its roots within the not-for-profit advocacy sector. IAVI developed out of a recognition within the global health and development field that more attention needed to be placed on discovering an AIDS vaccine; specifically one that can be successfully delivered to populations within those developing countries most significantly affected by the disease. IAVI has also been funded by donors associated with international development advocacy-type activities. First, by a traditional actor in the developing country health initiatives, the Rockefeller Foundation, and more recently by BMGF (which now also heavily funds science projects) as well as bilateral country donors such as UK's DfID. This has brought on board staff members with backgrounds and expertise in international development and public health, but who at the same time can work with scientists in both the public and commercial pharmaceutical sectors. A vice president of IAVI has claimed that this creates a 'clash of cultures' which influences the way IAVI's activities progress. This is the second interrelated factor that influences the way IAVI works as an integrator and/or broker and how these roles have changed over time. Increasingly, the staff numbers have been bolstered by those from a business background, which appears to have corresponded with the move towards greater efficiency and the streamlining of in-house research. The key strengths and weaknesses of organizations such as IAVI are presented in Box 10.3 below.

Box 10.3 Strengths of partnerships such as IAVI.

- Combining the best of many partners (e.g. government, private sector, the not-for-profit/third sector, and academia) bringing out competitiveness, efficiency, responsiveness, accountability, etc.
- Reducing regulation and other costs associated with product development and delivery
- Substantial financial bases
- Potential problems/weaknesses

- High costs of managing the partnership and keeping partner interests in agreement (e.g. clash of cultures problem)
- Difficulties in evaluating impact of such partnerships
- Limited control over health systems and other contextual factors in recipient communities

In this chapter we have used the IAVI case study to explore the complex evolutionary process towards developing and delivering effective technological solutions to a specific global health challenge. From a TM perspective, it has demonstrated the efforts made to combine interdisciplinary approaches and collaborative institutional arrangements to bridge the gap between clinical and basic science. The case has revealed the important roles and influences of the dynamics within the intervention area (HIV/AIDS in this case), the organizational histories and cultures, as well as the local contextual realities around disease burden, patient awareness, and institutional arrangements. IAVI has used a combination of historical and organizational attributes to package a response that has been seen to be working well within the reality of constrained health systems and an elusive vaccine target.

References

1. Chataway, J., Brusoni, S., Cacciatori, E., Hanlin, R., and Orsenigo, L., (2007). The International AIDS Vaccine Initiative (IAVI) in a changing landscape of vaccine development: a public private partnership as knowledge broker and integrator, *European Journal of Development Research*, **19**(1), pp. 100–117.
2. Kalua, F.A., Awotedu, A., Kamwanja, L.A., and Saka, J.D.K., eds. (2009). *Science, Technology and Innovation for Public Health in Africa*. Monograph, NEPAD Office of Science and Technology, Pretoria, Republic of South Africa.
3. Chataway, J., Hanlin, R., Mugwagwa, J., and Muraguri, L. (2010). Global health social technologies: Reflections on evolving theories and landscapes, *Research Policy*, **39**, pp. 1277–1288.
4. Cockburn, I.M., Henderson, R., and Stern, S. (1999). The diffusion of science driven drug discovery: organisational change in pharmaceutical research. *NBER Working Paper*, No. W7359.

5. Gambardella, A. (1995). Science and Innovation in the US Pharmaceutical Industry. *Cambridge University Press, Cambridge.*
6. Cockburn, I.M. and Henderson, R.M. (1998). Absorptive capacity, co-authoring behavior, and the organization of research in drug discovery. *Journal of Industrial Economics* **46**(2), pp. 157–182.
7. Kettler, H.E. and Towse, A. (2002). Public Private Partnerships for Research and Development: medicines and vaccines for diseases of poverty. *Office of Health Economics, London.*
8. Galambos, L. and Sturchio, J. (1998). Pharmaceutical firms and the transition to biotechnology: a study in strategic innovation. *Business History Review* **72**, pp. 250–278.
9. IAVI (2006). *Imagine a World without AIDS: The History of the International AIDS Vaccine Initiative.* IAVI, New York.
10. Skolnik, R. (2003). *An Independent Evaluation of the International AIDS Vaccine Initiative,* IAVI April. Available on the IAVI website: www.iavi.org.
11. Buse, K. and Walt, G. (2000). Global public–private partnerships: Part I: a new development in health? *Bulletin of the World Health Organization* **8**(4), pp. 549–561.
12. Lob-Levyt, J. (2008). Delivering the promise through new markets, new money and new partnerships for development. *Statement by Executive Secretary, GAVI Alliance,* available at http://www.gavialliance.org/media centre/statements/.
13. Chataway, J.C. and Smith J. (2006). The International AIDS Vaccine Initiative (IAVI): is it getting new science and technology to the world's neglected majority? *World Development* **34**(1), pp. 16–30.
14. Brinkerhoff, D. and Brinkerhoff, M. (2004). Partnerships between international donors and non-governmental development organisations: opportunities and constraints. *International Review of Administrative Sciences* **70** (2), pp. 253–270.
15. Saad, M., Rowe, K., and James, P. (1999). Developing and sustaining effective partnerships through a high level of trust. In: *Montanheiro, L., et al. eds., Public and Private Sector Partnerships: Furthering Development.* SHU Press, Sheffield.
16. Smith, R. (2000). Vaccines and medicines for the world's poorest: Public–private partnerships seem to be essential, *BMJ. 2000* April 8; **320**(7240), pp. 952–953.
17. Moran, M., Diaz, J., Garrison, C., Guzman, J., and Ropars, A. (2005). *The New Landscape of Neglected Disease Drug Development.* Wellcome Trust, London School of Economics and Political Science, London.

18. GAVI Alliance (2008). Progress Report, available on http://www.gavialliance.org/resources/2008_GAVI_Alliance_Progress_Report.pdf.
19. Elias, C. (2006). Can we ensure health is within reach for everyone? *Lancet* **368**, pp. S40–S41.
20. IAVI (2008). AIDS Vaccine blueprint 2008. A challenge to the field, a roadmap for progress. *The International AIDS Vaccine Initiative.*
21. IAVI (2008). The Innovation Fund Fact Sheet, available on http://www.iavi.org/Lists/IAVIPublications/attachments/2b9e821b-6800-43ef-8ccb-8ab57e2e8123/IAVI_Annual_Report_2008_ENG.pdf.
22. IAVI Press Release (2008). Mayor Bloomberg and Other Honourees Herald Opening of IAVI's New Design Lab. *IAVI Press Release. IAVI, New York*, http://www.iavi.org/viewfile.cfm?fid=49836 (accessed 15 March 2009).
23. DiMaggio, P.J. and Powell, W.W. (1983). The iron cage revisited: Institutional isomorphism and collective rationality in organisational fields. *American Sociological Review* **48**; pp. 147–160.
24. Vaughan, D. (2002). Signals and interpretive work: the role of culture in a theory of practical action. In: Karen Cerulo, Ed., *Culture in Mind: Toward a Sociology of Culture and Cognition*. Routledge, New York.

Part 5

Conclusions

Chapter 11

Is Translational Medicine the Future of Therapy?

Christopher-Paul Milne[a,*] **and James Mittra**[b,*]

[a]*Center for the Study of Drug Development, Tufts University Medical School, 75 Kneeland St., Suite 1100, Boston, MA 02111, USA*
[b]*ESRC Innogen Centre/STIS, University of Edinburgh, Old Surgeons' Hall, High School Yards, Edinburgh EH1 1LZ, UK*
*christopher.milne@tufts.edu, james.mittra@ed.ac.uk

11.1 What Does the Future Hold for Translational Medicine?

If translational medicine (TM) is the future of therapy, as the chapters in this book suggest, what might this future look like? Changing a research paradigm that has remained substantially unchanged for 50 years will no doubt require considerable time, money, effort, and leadership. Nevertheless, there is reason to believe that TM is more than just wishful thinking and will have staying power in the precarious world of scientific mood swings and the pendulum of investor and institutional funding cycles and scythes. It has become enmeshed with the evolutionary sweep of precompetitive collaboration, biomarkers, pharmacogenomics, and

Translational Medicine: The Future of Therapy
Edited by James Mittra and Christopher-Paul Milne

ISBN 978-981-4316-99-6 (Hardback), 978-981-4364-84-3 (eBook)
www.panstanford.com

personalized medicines, which will enable the incipient movement from population-based to patient-centered target markets [1]. In this final chapter, we reflect on the future of TM in the context of a broken R&D paradigm and the impetus toward patent-centered healthcare. We also discuss TM in the global context before drawing some final conclusions about the future of the field.

11.2 Fixing the R&D Paradigm

Investigator-initiated trials (IIT), often conducted at academic medical centers (AMCs), have long been recognized as playing a significant role in supporting TM studies that industry does not consider sufficiently economical to do itself [2]. Now that industry realizes that its current R&D model is broken, as many of the chapters in this book have highlighted, recognition of the role academia can play in "risk-sharing" the innovation process has flourished into two key movements. First, academic science/translational medicine centers are positioning themselves as early stage development modules and partners for pharmaceutical companies. Second, industry has developed an increased appetite for collaboration with academic centers. In fact, according to Garret A. FitzGerald, M.D., associate dean for translational research at the Raymond and Ruth Perelman School of Medicine at the University of Pennsylvania and director of the school's Institute for Translational Medicine and Therapeutics, the role of TM is to break with past practices in which the biomedical research industry has developed new drugs within a single company, and instead is increasing collaborations across academia and between pharmaceutical and biotechnology companies.

However, there are a few developmental problems: industry appears to be more willing to collaborate and risk-share with academia than academia is prepared to with industry; incentives and rewards for academic institutions are not aligned with those within industry; and there is a major gap in skills, ways of working, and business mediation and expertise that needs to be filled [3]. There have also been many practical problems in setting up collaborations, such as when contracts between industry and academia are delayed due to negotiations around intellectual property rights. The waxing and waning of conflict-of-interest rules frustrate industry when too rigid and worry watchdogs when they are too lax. Ethical review by different AMCs, sometimes in different countries, can cause problems with delays and inconsistency, on the one hand, or claims of lack of transparency on the other hand [4]. The challenges of public–private partnerships were illustrated in Chapter 9.

Yet, there are solutions in place that appear to be directed at the soft spots in the current R&D framework, especially open science initiatives exemplified by the Oncology Biomarker Qualification Initiative with $6.27m from approximately 10 companies and $3.75m from the NIH's National Cancer Institute in the United States. Another example is an education and training program, supported by the Wellcome Trust and 7 big pharma firms, to address the MD-researcher shortage at UK universities.

In addition to TM providing academia with funding opportunities from external sources through partnerships with the private sector, there is a promising trend in terms of its capacity to attract grant funding, mostly from the public sector (see Fig. 11.1).

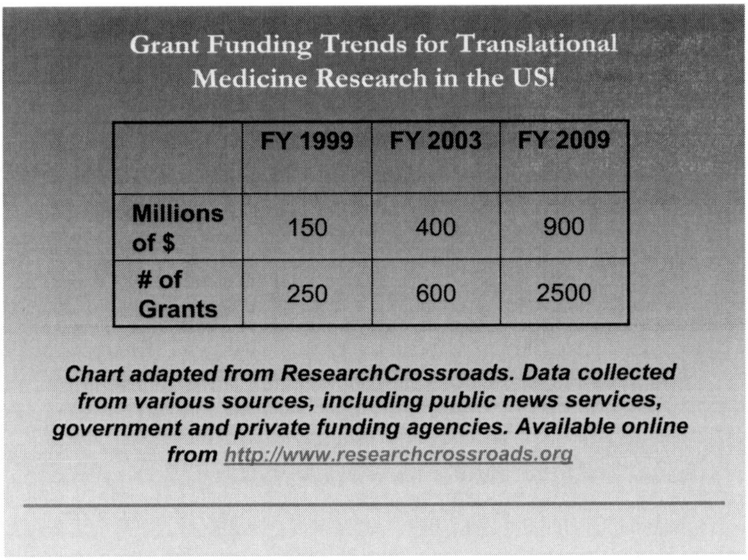

	FY 1999	FY 2003	FY 2009
Millions of $	150	400	900
# of Grants	250	600	2500

Figure 11.1 Grant funding trends for translational medicine research in the United States.

Although the number of grants increased 10-fold over a decade in the United States, an impressive rate of growth, the overall dollar amount remains relatively small at approximately $1bn in the latest year for which we have data. This was during a decade in which $1 trillion was spent on life sciences R&D in United States. In fact, it has been reported that the NIH has spent only 2% of its $40bn budget on translational research [5].

Obviously, academia will need to diversify its sources of funding. One way it has already found to do just that is by meeting the need for training and degree programs in interdisciplinary education in general, and TM in particular. In the current economic downturn, which is expected to last for several more years at the very least in the mature economies, there is likely to be continued and even growing interest in such programs. There are a number of examples of this: MD–PhD programs at many universities in translational research; Master's programs and 1-year certificates in clinical and translational sciences; and Master's of Medical Programs for science PhDs to name a few. The NIH has recognized both the need and the opportunity to take action and ensure the next generation of scientists has the resources and training necessary to translate scientific discoveries into new treatments as quickly and efficiently as possible. With this goal in mind, new NIH programs and groups are focusing on research workforce needs and how best to translate new findings into practice. The NIH has formed a Biomedical Research Workforce Working Group to develop a diverse, sustainable research workforce that will be prepared to advance new scientific discoveries into treatments. The working group is currently identifying the types of research positions that will help advance biomedical and behavioral sciences, as well as the kinds of transitional training and skills researchers need to have. In the future, new training models might include more opportunities for medical students and residents to explore clinical and translational research, as well as more programs designed to teach students how to carry out research effectively. The working group is expected to make recommendations to the NIH's Advisory Committee to the Director on how to build a sustainable and diverse research workforce that reflects the growing need for translational science [6].

11.3 Patient-Centered Healthcare

In concert with this growing momentum in the public sector, many major pharma companies have formed TM units with the broad goal to create a more direct connection between basic research and patient care. One way they have enhanced capacity to do this has been through collaboration with AMCs, as discussed above. Another way, however, is to conduct first-in-man studies earlier in the development process of a promising compound, by using healthy volunteers instead of patients, and testing efficacy through experiments instead of time and resource consuming clinical trials. For example, there is an experimental medicine TM consortium working on, among other projects, an anxiety challenge study artificially created in a laboratory setting in which the responses of volunteers to a putative therapeutic agent are being analyzed. TM is also riding the rising wave of several lucrative business segments for which it is both a purchaser and provider of products and services, as discussed in Chapter 3. This trend is predicted to increase over the coming decade as the markets for biomarkers, bioinformatics, and bioimaging both expand on their own and intersect with new business models generated by emerging markets for personalized medicine. The range of such technologies, and their potential role in future therapy, were comprehensively discussed in Chapters 6, 7, and 8.

Clearly, the forces of TM and patient-centered medicine are complementary, and payers are also driving the adoption of this concept and approach to healthcare delivery. Philosophically, they favor an approach called the Medical Home concept, which is a holistic approach, that focuses on the whole patient rather than a specific disease or organ. The emphasis is on personalized care and decision-making by patients in partnership with their physician. On the practical side, payers are requiring evermore "proof of value" through cost-effectiveness research (CER) and patient-reported outcomes (PRO) on both new and standard treatments, which in turn can be utilized to better inform the researchers further upstream about what works, what does not work, and what is still needed to fill gaps in clinical knowledge. In the early

2000s, Dr. Elias Zerhouni, then head of the NIH, expanded the definition of TM beyond "bench-to-bedside" to include the goal of patient-oriented and population research, which facilitates the efficient translation of new discoveries for use in the community. The plan for implementation of these efforts was detailed in the NIH Roadmap, and included the launching, in 2006, of the Clinical and Translational Science Award (CTSA) program [7]. As of the end of 2011, some 60 CTSA-funded academic centers had been established. One of the key areas of support provided to CTSA centers is access to translational technologies and resources such as mass spectrometry, imaging, ultrasound, positron emission tomography, gene expression, proteomics and translational cell, and gene therapies.

Looking forward, the fate of TM hangs in the balance as Congress and the President consider its future. The newly proposed and somewhat controversial National Center for Advancing Translational Sciences (NCATS) will focus on linking basic science research with new treatments and clinical care, as well as strengthening collaborations between the biomedical industry and academia. The controversy stems from the fact that NCATS will reorganize the NIH's National Center for Research Resources (NCRR), which houses the CTSA program. Under the NCATS proposal, the CTSAs would transfer to NCATS; while other NCRR programs would move to other institutes [6]. Currently, investment in TM research is estimated at $7–8bn per year in the United States with approximately $6bn of that funding coming from venture capital, $500m from angel investors, and only $750m from NIH. By itself, this seems like an impressive amount of funding. However, when compared to the $48bn spent on basic research and the $65bn spent on clinical development [8], or the $140bn spent annually on health care in the United States (see Fig. 11.2), it is relatively paltry. NCATS would establish a pivotal beach head for TM by providing a stable funding source for programs, education, and infrastructure.

In Europe, the R&D community has embraced the concept of TM and focused its attention on its main tools: biomarkers, bioimaging, and bioinformatics. In 2007, the EMA's Final Report from its Think Tank on Innovative Drug Development Approaches included a section on *Translational Medicine, Biomarkers/Surrogate Endpoints,*

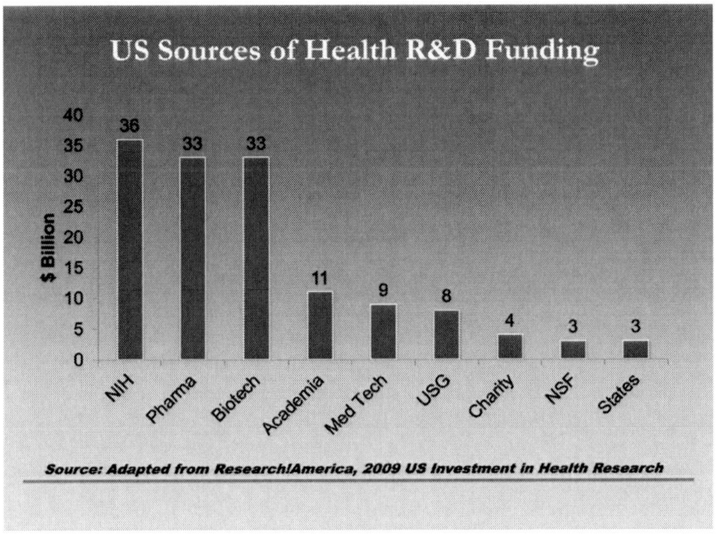

Figure 11.2 US sources of health R&D funding.

New Imaging Techniques and called for global collaboration from all sectors to move the field forward [9]. More recently, a call to action for bioinformatics was highlighted in the 4th Call for Proposals by the Innovative Medicines Initiative (IMI), at the 2011 World of Health IT in Budapest. Bioinformatics was featured in one of the three clusters of the 4th Call under the *EU Medical Information System*. It included a proposal for the creation of a European Translational Research Infrastructure & Knowledge Management Services (eTRIKS), in recognition that the continuous information sharing between pre-clinical and clinical activities needed by translational research is often inhibited by knowledge management obstacles related to access, management, integration, and analytics across diverse data types [10].

Looking forward once again, under the Seventh Framework Programme for Research and Technological Development (FP7), the European Commission's budget has committed to funding translational research until 2013 to open up clearly defined routes through which new products can come to the market unencumbered from developmental bottlenecks along the way. The long-term horizon of TM is likely tied to the fate of the newly created European Advanced

Translational Research Infrastructure in Medicine (EATRIS), one of the priority infrastructure projects in the roadmap of the European Strategy Forum on Research Infrastructure (ESFRI) and also funded by FP7. In an early stage development meeting, it was noted that funding and access to research infrastructure are critical to successfully transition from ideas to innovative products. The forum aims to bridge the lab and clinic by providing cross-disciplinary translational centers and fostering collaborations across Europe [11].

While patient-centered research is apparently headed on a somewhat separate trajectory from TM in Europe, it is very much a vibrant movement. For example, the National Institute for Health Research within the UK's NHS recently established the Academic Health Science Centres to integrate research, teaching, and clinical under a unified governance model to improve patient outcomes. A prominent feature of these Academic Health Science Centres is a Patient Advisory Board that seeks to identify problems, concerns, and weaknesses, as well as offer suggestions to improve the quality of clinical care.

11.4 The Geography of Change

While TM was firmly established in the United States and Europe by the middle of the last decade, it is still in an embryonic stage of development in the Asia-Pacific region. Nevertheless, it is becoming increasingly recognized as integral to domestic biopharmaceutical innovation. In Japan, present initiatives constitute more of a patchwork rather than any coordinated effort, even where it would appear otherwise. For example, the Ministry of Education, Science, Culture, and Sports in Japan oversees five university translational research centers, each with its own research activities in a variety of different areas. Despite this, attempts to better coordinate activity among centers have been slow, and linkages with the country's biopharmaceutical sector have been scarce [12].

In other parts of the Asia-Pacific region, however, some coordinated efforts are beginning to emerge, but they still remain small in number. One example is a joint initiative between the Agency for Science, Technology, and Research of Singapore (A*STAR) and the Health Research Council of New Zealand (HRC). The more than $2.4m fund, which is equally financed by both agencies, will provide grants for research in metabolic diseases and cancer. In Australia, for example, the Cooperative Research Centre for Biomarker Translation is a public–private partnership that aims to integrate TM concepts and techniques into a system already strong in basic R&D and early-stage clinical development. Taiwan boasts its own version of the United States inspired Critical Path Institute, and Singapore's Biomedical Science Initiative has declared that a goal of phase two of the program is "strengthening capabilities in translational and clinical research," following an initial phase of infrastructure development.

Popular with the public and publicly funded, bioscience parks can offer an attractive and practical "bricks and mortar" nidus for domestic coordination of TM initiatives. In Singapore, for example, the Biopolis complex houses a mix of public and private entities across a range of research areas. Collaboration through regional organizations, such as the Association of Southeast Asian Nations, are likely to be an effective vehicle for rallying around common objectives and for more efficient utilization of individual country strengths [13].

While Asia-Pacific has focused on building TM capacity through organizational and physical infrastructure, other emerging market countries, such as Brazil, are focusing on building a TM capacity through education and training. The goal of the Second São Paulo Advanced School in Translational Sciences is to offer a scenario to discuss molecular medicine, from basic to translational aspects, in both cancer and neurodegenerative diseases. This is also an initiative of the Brazilian National Institute for Science and Technology in Oncogenomics (INCITO) and the National Institute for Translational Neuroscience (INNT). The programs bring together some of the world's foremost experts in the biology and treatment of these devastating diseases in an exceptional environment of learning and information sharing based on cutting-edge science. The School will offer excellent opportunities for networking to a new generation of scientists and will inspire them to pursue careers in translational research in cancer and neurodegenerative diseases.

TM therefore provides new territory for globalization, collaboration, and harmonization [14]. With the United States and Europe leading the way, TM may facilitate a "fast follower" effect among the Asia-Pacific region and emerging markets in the Americas toward a more efficient and effective global R&D enterprise.

11.5 The Future of Therapy

Although there is evidence to suggest TM has the tools to accomplish its goals, the TM trademark must avoid becoming just a new term for old process [2]. New treatments, diagnostics, preventatives, and modes of delivery must be developed while taking into account limitations in funding, infrastructure, and government's willingness-to-pay. These goals could be accomplished without a significant reordering of the biomedical enterprise or reallocation of resources, but through refocusing currently available intellectual and investment capital (e.g., patient advisory boards, CTSA partnering programs, or interdisciplinary graduate programs). Small changes across a variety of niches, including the regulatory regimes for new therapies, could have a large impact on the broader healthcare ecosystem [7]. Alternatively, we could shape-shift the R&D enterprise wholesale to make successful translation from "bench-to-bedside-and-back" the actual lynchpin in how we create new therapies, instead of the more conventional figurative box connecting basic and clinical research in some stylized but unrealized rendering of how the process ought to work. Such an undertaking would require relatively simultaneous changes at a number of different levels (see Box 11.1 below).

As we have discussed in the preceding chapters of this book, the challenge is as daunting as the need for change is tantalizing. All the authors who have contributed to this book have recognized and elucidated the many challenges facing contemporary R&D and patient healthcare delivery, as well as the opportunities and bottlenecks facing TM. They have covered this from the scientific, commercial, social, and regulatory angles, as well as explored regional differences and unique challenges for low-resource regions. The institutional dynamics of collaborative projects are just as

Box 11.1 What needs to happen? [15,16]

Interface — specifically, translational medicine research interfaces (TMRIs), to grow a virtual translational institute from seedbed of CTSA program to do: target ID and validation; IP crafting; business development; exploratory development plan; funding scouts; as well as provide intersection point for industry and government into incubator technology community

Individual — need to develop new professional with specific skills to navigate the interfaces and mitigate fragmentation

Institution — have to develop support structure to bring together different competencies relevant to TM that already exist within universities, i.e. where resources already exist, core competencies just need to be focused

International — globalization of component parts of process require initiative to form international network similar to TMRIs but on a global scale to ensure standardization of quality and ethical parameters and negotiate disparities in regulatory procedures, intellectual property rights (IPR), and financing

Incorporation — of social science factors such as socio-economic, behavior psychology, and ethics in order to address all three levels of TM barriers: bench-to-bedside; bedside-to-community (hospitals or medical specialty); community to policy (integration into diagnostic kits, standardized medical guidelines, or insurance reimbursement policies)

challenging as the scientific and technical challenges. The lack of an agreed definition of TM within policy circles and no formal evaluative criteria for TM projects, which was the focus of Chapter 5, highlights the continuing challenges that must be overcome.

The volume of data being generated in the biological and clinical arenas accumulates much faster than we can assimilate into a body of knowledge that can be utilized efficiently or effectively. TM's capacity to deal with the information overload (both in amount and heterogeneity), which was discussed in Chapter 8, will depend on assembling trans-disciplinary teams from various medical sciences as well as specialized "informaticians" to work alongside them to support analyses and develop new hypotheses in domain specific areas. Training programs and curricula that incorporate biotranslational informatics (BTI) concepts will accordingly become essential to redress the currently limited number of such informaticians capable of fabricating the linkages between biological and clinical silos through which paradigm shifting hypotheses may be elucidated.

Another important set of barriers are the current lack of accepted imaging standards, variability in platforms across multiple sites, and limited data sharing that continue to hamper imaging biomarker clinical translation and development. Chapter 7 presented the state-of-the-art in imaging technologies and highlighted how they may be used to drive the TM paradigm. Current available imaging biomarkers provide structural, physiological, and metabolic information. More novel and innovative imaging platforms come with great promise to annotate structure with molecular signatures that tightly link to the pathophysiology or to the therapeutic mechanism of action. These cutting edge modalities will reveal information on *in vivo* pharmacokinetics, receptor expression and occupancy, and/or molecular signaling, which will greatly enhance the precision and effectiveness for modern drug research & development. However, greater resource-sharing through pre-competitive collaboration among private and public sector scientists, as well as proactive engagement with regulatory agencies, is needed to coordinate, conduct, and stimulate research and education about the development, standardization, validation, and qualification of imaging biomarkers.

Despite the deluge of words anticipating the imminent arrival of the age of personalized medicine, changing a well-established behavior is generally difficult, particularly when the evidence base is underdeveloped and successful examples are few and far between. When first introduced, predictive genetic testing suffered from ill-defined clinical utility that lead to confusion and rejection by the practicing healthcare professionals. Translating results into patient care best practices is challenging in the absence of scientific consensus, as well as practitioner training and familiarity with what amounts to a new way of making decisions about appropriate care. There is also lingering apprehension about genomic medicine from the public due to privacy issues. These are more than just philosophical hurdles, however. There are practical barriers relating to the sensitivity, specificity, convenience, and cost of companion diagnostics, as well as the appropriate business models and value systems for developing therapies for stratified or personalized patient populations. There are currently no real regulatory or financial incentives for conducting pharmacogenomically enriched clinical trials, despite the potential gain in terms of process efficiency as well as product safety and efficacy. Insurance reimbursement and cost-effectiveness analyses are currently established from a health-care system perspective rather than from an individual patient perspective. Payers have demonstrated a somewhat underwhelming willingness-to-pay for the early fruits of the genomic revolution. Personalized medicine may be a great idea whose time has come, but whose bill has not found a willing payer!

What does this mean for TM? Clearly the vitality of the TM movement in the public sector, due to its interest in promoting patient-centered care, bodes well for its continued appeal to the commercial sector. From industry's perspective, there is a keen appreciation that a translational approach to R&D is key to efficiently taking advantage of breakthrough technology to achieve both better productivity and an improved pipeline of new products. As always, economics guides the direction of investment and resource commitment by industry and, less directly but just as implacably, by government. In the short term, the economics of TM and its budding business segments look attractive at a time when the economic environment in general looks less so. In the longer term, TM and personalized/stratified medicines, as well as associated tools and technologies, have the potential to re-energize flagging economic prospects for both the therapeutics and diagnostics business segments, as well as the R&D engines of academia. Subsequently, those responsible for health care delivery will have to pay their share for TM or face a future in which healthcare costs continue to escalate while patients' therapeutic options stagnate. Ultimately, TM will likely provide tomorrow's treatments, and perhaps cures, along an evolving innovation pathway whose outlines are perhaps only beginning to take shape today. Together, we hope the chapters in this book provide the reader a good, comprehensive overview of the key opportunities and challenges in the field of TM, from a broad range of perspectives, and spur further debate and reflection about the future of drug development and healthcare in a variety of international and institutional contexts.

References

1. Milne, C.-P. (2009). Can translational medicine bring us out of the R&D wilderness? *Personalized Medicine,* September, **6**(5), pp. 543–553.
2. Wehling, M. (2008). Translational medicine: science or wishful thinking? *Journal of Translational Medicine,* **6**(31) DOI:10.1186/1479-5876-6-31.
3. Bowe, C. (2011). Lost in translation — notes from the translational medicine undercurrent. *SCRIP,* newsletter, November 11.
4. Nicogossian, A., Grigoriev, A. I., Kloiber, O., Zimmerman, T., *et al.* (2010). Translational research, evidence-based medicine and medical policy, *World Medical & Health Policy* **2**(4), Article 1, available at: http://www.psocommons.org/wmhp/vol2/iss4/art1.
5. Duncan, D.E. (2010). How to reboot bioscience revolution, *CNN-Money.com,* October 13.
6. Mann, S. (2011). NIH prepares future workforce for translational science. *AAMC Reporter*: September.
7. Milne, C.-P. and Kaitin, K.I. (2009). Translational medicine: an engine of change for bringing new technology to community health. *Science Translational Medicine,* 4 November **1**(5) pp. 5 DOI: 10.1126/scitranslmed.3000222.
8. Milken Institute (Presentation) (2011). *Financial Innovations for Translational Research,* July 19.
9. Final report from the EMEA/CHMP-Think-Tank Group on Innovative Drug Development (2007). *Innovative Drug Development Approaches.* March 22, Doc. Ref. EMEA/127318/2007, London.
10. Piai, S. (2011). The Innovative Medicine Initiative launches its 4th call. Entry posted May 24, available at http://idc-insights-community.com/posts/8572000708.
11. EATRIS International Conference (2010). *From Basic Research to Medical Innovation,* conference report, October, Rome, Italy.

12. Fukushima, M. (2006). Translational research in Japan: opportunities and obstacles. *Clinical Evaluation*, **33**(3), pp. 499–503.
13. Wilson, A. and Milne, C.-P. (2009). The translational medicine movement in the Asia Pacific region. *Pharma Focus Asia* **12** pp. 30–32.
14. Meeting announcement, available at http://www.nature.com/natureevents/science/events/11458-S_o_Paulo_Advanced_School_in_Translational_Science.
15. Albani, S. and Prakken, B. (2009). The advancement of translational medicine—from regional challenges to global solutions. *Nature Medicine* **15** pp. 1006–1009. DOI:10.1038/nm0909-1006.
16. IBM Research. How translational medicine can improve health care, available at http://researcher.ibm.com/researcher/view_project.phy?id=1875.

Index